Trials of Labour

CRITICAL PERSPECTIVES ON PUBLIC AFFAIRS
Series Editors: Duncan Cameron and Daniel Drache

This series, sponsored by the Canadian Centre for Policy Alternatives and co-published by McGill-Queen's University Press, is intended to present important research on Canadian policy and public affairs. Books are by leading economic and social critics in the Canadian academic community and will be useful for classroom texts and the informed reader as well as for the academic specialist.

The Canadian Centre for Policy Alternatives promotes research on economic and social issues facing Canada. Through its research reports, studies, conferences, and briefing sessions, the CCPA provides thoughtful alternatives to the proposals of business research institutions and many government agencies. Founded in 1980, the CCPA holds that economic and social research should contribute to building a better society. The centre is committed to publishing research that reflects the concerns of women as well as men; labour as well as business; churches, cooperatives, and voluntary agencies as well as governments; disadvantaged individuals as well as those more fortunate. Critical Perspectives on Public Affairs will reflect this tradition through the publication of scholarly monographs and collections.

Trials of Labour

The Re-emergence of Midwifery

BRIAN BURTCH

McGill-Queen's University Press
Montreal & Kingston • London • Buffalo

© McGill-Queen's University Press 1994
ISBN 0-7735-1141-5 (cloth)
ISBN 0-7735-1143-1 (paper)

Legal deposit first quarter 1994
Bibliothèque nationale du Québec

Printed in Canada on acid-free paper

This book has been published with the help of a grant
from the Social Science Federation of Canada, using
funds provided by the Social Sciences and Humanities
Research Council of Canada.

Canadian Cataloguing in Publication Data

Burtch, Brian E., 1949–
  Trials of labour: the re-emergence of midwifery
  Includes bibliographical references and index.
  ISBN 0-7735-1141-5 (bound) –
  ISBN 0-7735-1143-1 (pbk.)
  1. Midwives – Canada. 2. Midwives – Legal status,
  laws, etc. – Canada. 3. Obstetrics – Canada.
  4. Obstetrics – Law and legislation – Canada. I. Title.
  RG950.B87 1994   618.2'0233   C93-090664-0

Typeset in Palatino 10/12
by Caractéra production graphique inc., Quebec City

*To Leora, Aymer, and Doreen Burtch
and
in memory of Diane Corkum, James Brown,
and the Gordons*

Contents

Figures

Tables

Acknowledgments

It would not have been possible for me to write this book without the cooperation and good faith of many midwives. Midwives practising in British Columbia, Saskatchewan, and Ontario provided birth records for the home birth study described in chapter four. Jocelan Coty inspired this topic for my doctoral research, and provided encouragement and support. Bob Ratner was a steady force and friend throughout this research, as were Neil Guppy and Helga Jacobson. Joan Anderson, Nancy Waxler-Morrison, John Hogarth, and David Coburn also made useful comments.

Alison Rice and Elaine Carty have been stalwarts in rethinking the nature of maternity and infant services. Stan Howard was a great help, along with others active with the Midwifery Task Force of British Columbia and the Midwives Association of British Columbia. The Law Foundation of British Columbia provided funds for an educational videotape, *Midwifery and the Law* (Simon Fraser University 1991). Many thanks to Keet Neville and Michael Doherty for their efforts in documenting the midwifery movement.

I am deeply grateful to a host of people who contributed to the research effort: Jean Lyons, Cheryl Anderson, Lee Saxell, Gale Lanthier, Gary Brown, Bruce Arnold, Charlene MacLellan, Carol-Anne Letty, Linda Knox, Vicki Van Wagner, Theo Dawson, Lauren Knoblauch, Barb Ray, Lynn McLean, Lesley Biggs, Cecilia Benoit, Richard Berger, Rampee Lidder, Nick Larsen, Jude Kornelsen, and Terry Meindl. Maureen Gabriel, Debbie Nickel, and Azima Buell were invaluable as research assistants in their careful attention to coding birth records, proofreading, and updating various tables. Paul Woodward prepared several of the figures that appear in the text. Sharon Rynders and Carla Hotel provided great help, including rescuing an entire chapter that I thought was lost to the ethers.

Considerable information was provided under the auspices of the Ontario Association of Midwives, the Midwives Association of British Columbia, the Midwives Association of Saskatchewan, and the Midwifery Task Force of British Columbia. Representatives of the International Confederation of Midwives and the Royal College of Midwives were also very helpful. I wish to thank the women whose documented births provided a clearer basis for discussing the nature of midwifery practice in Canada.

Carol Hird has been an inspirational companion who leads by example with her work in support of midwives worldwide. She has taught me how to burn the candle from three ends, not two. I wish to acknowledge my daughter Leora Burtch for her understanding during the writing of the book, and my parents Doreen and Aymer Burtch for their encouragement all these years.

The research was supported in part through a doctoral fellowship provided by the Social Sciences and Humanities Research Council of Canada. The council's assistance is gratefully acknowledged. This work was made possible through the support of the Social Sciences Federation of Canada, and the helpful comments of five anonymous reviewers who read earlier drafts of this work.

Mary Lynn Stewart and Arlene McLaren deserve credit for their encouragement and timely advice. I was very fortunate in having Philip Cercone, Joan McGilvray, Ann Quinn, and other staff of McGill-Queen's University Press assist with the development of this book. Thanks to Kathy Johnson for copy-editing the manuscript. To all the people mentioned above, and to others "between the lines" of this acknowledgment, thanks for your support.

Trials of Labour

CHAPTER ONE

The Midwifery Movement in Canada

Midwives were in demand among the settlers in Nova Scotia, for in 1755 a request came from Colonel Sutherland, in command at Lunenberg, for "two proper persons to reside there as midwives at a salary of two pounds a year, as the inhabitants were losing so many of their children."

Cited in Jan Gibbon and Mary Matthewson,
Three Centuries of Canadian Nursing

THE PROPER PERSON

Historically, midwives have been the traditional caregivers at births. Today, midwives attend the majority of births worldwide. They are established as an integral part of maternity and infant care in virtually every country in the world. In twentieth-century Canada, however, midwives nearly disappeared as "feminine networks" lost ground to the developing science of obstetrics (Mitchinson 1991, 164). The importance of midwifery was recognized in earlier times in Canada. Colonel Sutherland's request for midwives in eighteenth-century Nova Scotia reflects their importance. Midwives were active for thousands of years among the first peoples of North America, and were an esteemed part of settlements in America (Edwards and Waldorf 1984, 148) and colonial Canada, providing childbirth attendance and healing. A number of documents attest to the importance of lay midwives in coastal settlements in British Columbia and Newfoundland, the prairie region, and in urban centres during the eighteenth and nineteenth centuries (Benoit 1991, Biggs 1983).

The place of the community midwife in Canada has changed dramatically. With the very recent exceptions of Ontario and Alberta, Canada is alone among industrialized nations in not providing a distinct legal status for practising midwives. Once respected and sought after as a resource for settlers, community midwives in Canada have in recent years been subject to prosecution or other formal proceedings (such as coroner's inquests or inquiries). Whether one sees the Canadian midwife's status as *alegal* (having no clear status in law) or *illegal*, the past two decades of the midwifery movement in Canada confirm that midwives are liable to be charged with practising midwifery (or medicine) without a licence. Criminal prosecution of community midwives has also been carried out. Even where such formal prosecution is not launched, there have been numerous coroner's inquests and inquiries into midwifery practice, usually after infant deaths.

In this book I will examine the ways in which the midwife's role has been transformed throughout Canada. This transformation has been threefold: first, campaigns against midwifery practice have led to the near-eradication of the lay midwife; second, birth and pregnancy have been redefined as medical events, requiring the supervision of physicians and nurses and the virtually routine application of technological aids; third, midwifery was the subject of a complex series of responses in law and state policy, leaving only a limited footing for establishing midwifery as a self-regulating profession in Canada and the United States.

Trials of Labour traces the difficulties faced by midwives and their supporters in questioning the domination of birth care by physicians and nurses and the nearly complete management of labour, delivery, and early post-partum care in hospital settings. Yet this is not simply a story of victimization writ large: Canadian midwives have to date avoided criminal conviction, continue to lobby for legal recognition, and attend births even though midwifery is not clearly recognized in law. Nevertheless, it is ironic that midwives – who are entrenched in most other countries – have received a generally dismissive and sometimes hostile reaction from the dominant health professions and government bodies responsible for justice and health care. In the media and the courts, and in debates over birth care, midwives in Canada are often on a form of trial, their competence called into question and their motivations and practices subject to distortion.

Midwives seek to restore a sense of intimacy and community throughout the birth process. In this they face limitations, not all of them traceable to official resistance. Dramatic changes have occurred in family structures and communities in Canada and on a global scale. The family as the locus of childbirth and child-rearing has become diffuse, with institutions such as the hospital, the school, and child-care centres taking more responsibility and control. The sense of community has also been altered, particularly in terms of a community of women. Historically, women formed communities of interest that included pregnancy, childbirth, and health care (Ehren-reich and English 1973; Oakley 1976, 17–58). These communities thrived well into this century in some regions of Canada. Outport villages in Newfoundland are one example of the importance of midwives and the community of women (Benoit 1991). Kitzinger (1978: 125–6) adds that midwives in peasant societies had high pres-tige and considerable power as birth attendants, and for presiding over the forces of fertility. Structural changes in midwifery, families, and communities are thus central to an understanding of midwifery practice in health care systems.

The professionalization of midwifery – such that pregnant women are made into clients, and served by midwives, nurses, and physi-cians – is a major force shaping the midwifery movement. In a sense, while this ideology of professionalism is a barrier to midwifery, it has also given life to the modern midwifery movement. Professional management of birth, enjoying a near-hegemonic status in North America (with approximately 99 per cent of births occurring in hos-pitals or clinics under professional management), has been subject to wide criticism for its depersonalized care and excessive interven-tion, and at times for the iatrogenic effects of medical or nursing supervision of birth. Illich (1977: 35–36) describes *clinical iatrogenesis* as "all clinical conditions for which remedies, physicians, or hospitals are the pathogens, or 'sickening' agents."

Criticism of obstetrical procedures ranges from a growing feminist literature that regards some procedures as reproducing the domi-nance of technology and professional needs over women's bodies and interests, to ongoing criticism from medical and nursing practitioners concerning high caesarean section rates and other forms of "tech-nocratic interference in the process of childbirth" (Cohen and Estner 1983, 11). Concerns over morbidity associated with modern obstetrics in Canada and elsewhere have been expressed in the medical pro-fession. Some physicians have involved themselves in support of midwifery: these include Cheryl Anderson, Kirsten Emmott, Bernd Wittmann, Gabor Mate, Murray Enkin (Canada), Marsden Wagner (World Health Organization), G.J. Kloosterman (Netherlands), and Wendy Savage (United Kingdom). This list is far from comprehensive, but highlights support for midwifery within the medical community. While acknowledging the importance of specialized interventions and various forms of monitoring for high-risk births and in the care of premature infants, these physicians see great value in restoring birth management to the care of midwives.

The midwifery debate in Canada is also discussed in the context of other health-care systems. This requires an appreciation of the political economy of health care. While the majority of births worldwide are attended by midwives (Kitzinger 1988, 9), there are substantial disparities in resources and training of birth attendants among nations. In Canada, the United States, and the United Kingdom, over 90 per cent of births are attended by medically trained personnel, including midwives. Within these countries, disparities in care available to women and in infant mortality (especially among the poor) are evident. The promise of medically supervised births thus has its failings in practice, whether owing to an erosion of birth-related knowledge among expectant women, unnecessary interventions, or inadequate access by needy women to services such as prenatal care (see Mitford 1992, 219). In contrast, India, Malaysia, and several African countries report less than 30 per cent of births attended by such trained workers. Whereas many developing countries lack skilled birth care, in wealthier countries "growing disenchantment with modern medicine's approach to birth care is leading to a resurgence of midwifery" (Seager and Olson 1986, section 11).

DEFINITIONS OF MIDWIFERY

There are many definitions of midwifery. A generic definition of "midwifery" includes anyone, male or female, who assists a woman in childbirth, including certified nurse-midwives, community midwives, folk or lay midwives, neighbours and spouses who assist at birth, obstetricians, general practitioners, obstetrical nurses, and those compelled to assist at unexpected births (such as police officers and paramedics). A more restrictive definition of midwifery includes only female birth attendants. In this usage, "wife" (originally "wyfe," or woman) and "woman" are linked. There is some debate over whether the term "midwife" includes *all* women who are present with the mother at birth, or only "a woman by whose means the delivery is effected" (*Oxford English Dictionary*).

THERE IS CONSIDERABLE agreement that midwives form an occupational grouping; this means that occasional participants in birth are not correctly defined as midwives. The midwife is thus "any individual who, by choice, assists a woman in the process of delivering her baby, and who consciously assumes some degree of responsibility for the health and well-being of mother and child. This is the broadest possible definition, and includes trained nurse-midwives, traditional midwives or birth attendants in all cultures, as well as trained obstetricians. *It also includes men and women who together decide to deliver their child at home.* It excludes firemen, policemen, emergency service personnel and random individuals who fortuitously deliver an occasional baby as the result of idiosyncratic circumstances" (Cobb 1981, 75, emphasis added).

Many midwives see midwifery as distinct from medical specialties and general practice. For them, this incorporation of midwifery and obstetrics is misleading. It obscures significant differences in practice and philosophy between midwives and other birth attendants. This is especially so in that it is thought that midwives should honour women's preferences in birth, and that midwives should establish a deep rapport with expectant mothers and families, partly through intensive prenatal care.

In Canada, two forms of midwifery practice were prominent in the 1970s and 1980s. As we will see later, these forms are no longer cut-and-dried: midwives increasingly are seeking multiple routes of entry to the midwifery profession. The first was community or independent midwifery, associated primarily with home birth, as well as labour coaching in hospital, prenatal classes, and lobbying government to restore midwifery. The second form was more closely associated with obstetrical nursing, termed *nurse-midwifery*. Advocates of the nurse-midwife pointed to the versatility, training, and public appeal of birth attendants who were also qualified as nurses.

Community midwives in Canada have an uncertain and precarious status in law. They may be disadvantaged without the established professional and legal protections accorded physicians and nurses. Community midwives prize continuity of care with their clients, from regular prenatal visits (usually of longer duration that that of general practitioners), care through labour and delivery, and follow-up via post-partum visits with the mother and family. By the early 1980s in British Columbia, however, most community midwives were not licensed midwives, nor did they have access to formal training. Community midwives were thus largely self-taught, referring to available texts and other materials, as well as apprenticing with other, more experienced midwives. Since the early 1980s, with the advent of a midwifery school in Vancouver, many of these community midwives have completed an academic and clinical program in midwifery, and have been accredited as midwives through Washington state. This accreditation means that the midwives can practise in Washington state or in other jurisdictions with reciprocity. Initially, British Columbia did not provide reciprocity, so the midwives could not establish lawful practices in the province.

The term "community midwife" is more popular than "lay midwife." "Lay midwife" is thought to connote inferiority and dangerousness. Many community midwives have nursing training, hospital experience, and accreditation. Unlike obstetrical nurses, who practise in hospital settings or other accredited sites, community midwives in British Columbia practise for the most part out-of-hospital. This practice includes primary prenatal and postnatal care and assistance with home births. Community midwives may also provide birth control counselling, advice on breastfeeding, prenatal classes, and labour coaching in hospital. Community midwives, once thriving in various parts of Canada, have generally been discouraged from practice. In Vancouver, for example, approximately twenty community midwives in 1980 and fifteen in 1993 were known to be practising, despite significant population growth in greater Vancouver.

A nurse-midwife is a birth attendant who has completed nursing training, is registered with the local (or national, state, or provincial) nursing association, and has completed additional midwifery training in an accredited program. The term "nurse-midwifery" is to a large extent an Americanism. In many other jurisdictions, midwifery is not seen as a hyphenated profession. Some argue that nurse-midwifery keeps midwives on a lower rung of the hierarchy and under physician control of one form or another. Supporters of the concept point to the legacy of nursing care, and to considerable evidence that nurse-midwives have earned the trust of the women they care for. The sphere of practice of certified nurse-midwives (CNMs) can be very broad. Nurse-midwifery may involve continuity of care beyond attendance at labour and delivery:

[The certified nurse-midwife] might be employed by a hospital, by a medical center, by an affiliated community-based maternal and child health service, or by an obstetrician-midwife group practice. She manages the complete maternity care for mothers with an essentially normal course of pregnancy. She always functions with readily available medical consultation should any sudden medical complications arise. Today's modern midwife is prepared to function in all areas of [a] woman's health maintenance concerned with reproductive processes, including family planning and childbirth. Perinatal care and newborn health management are integral parts of midwifery practice (Lang 1979, 145).

Lang's definition encapsulates several major themes concerning the redefinition of midwifery in contemporary medical care. First, the CNM is often not an independent practitioner working out of her home or private office. She usually works as an employee or a partner in a practice. Levy and his associates (1971, 51) reported that "nurse-midwives are never independent practitioners; they always function within the framework of a physician-directed health service." This assumption of the subordination of nursing deserves critical scrutiny, for it underestimates the role of the nursing profession in maternity and infant care. A second theme is that non-medical personnel (such as lay midwives) are excluded from the CNM's network of collaborating birth attendants. Third, the premise of "readily available" medical consultation obscures the very tangible conflicts between the sphere of practice of nurse-midwives and that of other birth attendants. Rooks and Fischman (1980, 990) saw nursing training as an integral part of the development of American midwifery. The International Federation of Gynaecology and Obstetrics (FIGO), together with the International Confederation of Midwives (ICM), formulated a widely accepted definition of midwifery that encompasses nurse-midwifery and other forms of midwifery (see Phaff et al. 1975, 2).

A midwife is a person who, having been regularly admitted to a midwifery education program, duly recognized in the country in which it is located, has successfully completed the prescribed course of studies in midwifery and has acquired the requisite qualifications to be registered and/or legally licensed to practice midwifery. She must be able to give the necessary supervision, care and advice to women during pregnancy, labour and the postpartum period, to conduct deliveries on her own responsibility and to care for the newborn and the infant. This care includes preventive measures, the detection of abnormal conditions in mother and child, the procurement of medical assistance and the execution of emergency services in the absence of medical help.

She has an important task in health counselling and education, not only for the women but also within the family and the community. The work should involve antenatal education and preparation for parenthood and extends to certain areas of gynaecology, family planning and child care. She may practice in hospitals, clinics, health units, domiciliary conditions or any other service.

This broad definition of the midwife's role has been accepted in many countries. The potentially wide sphere of practice for midwives contrasts with the artificial division of Canadian midwives into the more independent but illegal practice of community midwifery or the hospital-based employment of nurses trained in midwifery. In fact, there is a considerable blurring of these two kinds of midwifery, such that the generic term *midwife* is now widely used in Canada. "Midwife" is a stand-alone term in most other nations.

Obstetrical nurses are legal practitioners under the British Columbia Registered Nurses Act. Nevertheless, their legal status has been accompanied by the containment of midwifery skills within many obstetrical settings. As discussed in chapter two, the FIGO/ICM definition may be compromised when midwifery services are implemented so as to restrict what midwives can legitimately do as caregivers. For a critique of the doctrine that midwives *must* be nurses, see Flint (1986a).

The contrived distinction of nurses versus midwives has been questioned by the midwifery movement in Canada, the United States, and other countries. The midwifery movement in North America draws on community midwives, nurses and nurse-midwives, and supporters of midwifery. While there is some disagreement over the proper sphere of midwifery practice in Canada, those active in the movement have generally held fast to the principle that midwifery ought to be legalized. This would mean that midwives would no longer be singled out as objects of highly publicized, expensive legal proceedings. The midwifery movement also espouses public education, holding that there is support among the public for midwifery attendance. "Midwife" is thus seen as a more inclusive term, to be applied to those who are expert in the management of normal childbirth, and to those who assist in high-risk management supervised by medical specialists. The movement to bolster midwifery in Canada thus draws on a range of practitioners and supporters, and seeks to establish means of certification, training, guidelines for practice, and a more collegial relationship with other practitioners.

THE MIDWIFERY CONTROVERSY

The modern controversy over reinstating midwifery services in Canada is best understood in the light of conventional research surrounding maternity and infant care and a growing body of critical literature addressing the nature of power and control in health services and social life generally. In this book I will provide an argument in support of the reinstatement of midwifery in Canada, an argument that is well supported through conventional studies of birthing services. The hegemonic powers of the medical profession and formal state powers (in legislation and social policy) have generally served to curb and weaken initiatives for the reinstatement of midwifery services across Canada. The short history of the modern midwifery movement in Canada confirms the potential danger of compromising midwifery by granting it legal status at the considerable price of imposing medical direction upon it.

Much contemporary research on childbirth has been medically oriented, addressing obstetrical techniques and birth outcomes. This approach is directed toward improved services for women in labour and their infants. It is associated with considerable improvements in the management of high-risk pregnancies and methods of treating newborns suffering from low birth weight, genetic deformities, fetal alcohol syndrome, and the like. Technical discussions of the prevention and treatment of mortality and morbidity are central to this literature, along with a growing interest in health promotion for expectant mothers and infants. This literature is of course valuable, and arguably invaluable, in understanding the mechanics and problems associated with childbearing.

Other approaches to childbirth present a less clinical or technical portrait of childbirth. For instance, sociological studies of pregnancy and childbirth have shown interest in the history of birthing practices in North America and elsewhere and in cross-cultural variations in birth (Oakley 1980). A vast literature has emerged on the high rates of intervention in western obstetrics and ongoing work suggests that procedures could be modified such that morbidity might be lessened without compromising the well-being of mothers of infants. There has been little information on the self-regulation of birth attendants by professional associations such as colleges of physicians and surgeons and nursing colleges, or on the more direct involvement of the legal apparatus of the state. Framed within the research and clinical experience of modern medicine and nursing, North American perspectives on birth have recently broadened. This broadening includes an appreciation of other countries where midwifery is much more integrated with medicine and nursing. Proponents of this critical approach thus see midwifery and health promotion as cut from the same cloth. Midwives can promote public health and provide a valued service if the health system allows for qualified midwifery instruction and practice.

The anomalous situation of midwives in Canada – at best, alegal; at worst, subject to inquests, inquiries, trials, and penalties – stems from a complex mixture of medical ideology, repressive criminal legislation, and protective civil legislation in the form of medical acts. Those medical acts grant substantial powers to medical associations in the supervising of and intervening in the birth process. For midwives, the renewed interest in theories of the state in western capitalist societies provides a framework for understanding the resistance to re-establishing midwifery, and also charts directions that may lead to the broadening of options in maternity and infant care. Specifically, the central question is how state intervention in childbirth attendance in British Columbia has contributed to the outlaw status of the midwifery profession. These questions are discussed in more detail in chapter five.

Critical theory begins with the assumption that the state secures patterns of domination and subordination in Canada and elsewhere. The nature of domination encompasses patterns of male dominance over women (as employees and patients) within the medical and other spheres, the everyday power of professionals over non-professionals, and the spectrum of routine technological intervention in childbirth. State support for the medicalization of childbirth is historically rooted in a legal monopoly of practice for male physicians and surgeons. The monopoly status protected the interests of the then emergent, now dominant, medical profession. The exclusion of non-medical practitioners by the state thus enabled medical practices to develop with limited competition from "irregular" practitioners (Biggs 1983; Mitchinson 1991).

The midwifery movement, as a public interest force, challenges the assumption that the state has acted in the public interest by promoting a virtual monopoly for physicians and nurses in managing births. In its general non-responsiveness, or its active prosecution of midwives, the state has often been complicit in the historical takeover of birth attendance. As mentioned earlier, the takeover is almost complete: close to 100 per cent of births in North America involve hospital-based deliveries supervised by medical personnel (Arms 1977; Tonkin 1981).

Government officials are not presented as simply in league with medical interests in Canada. There is a degree of autonomy exercised by officials in reconsidering social policies. Conspiracy theories of the state and health professions oversimplify the complexity of the midwifery debate and the prospects for new policies for midwifery in Canada.

This book also examines the practices of community midwives. Reference is made to my study of 1,006 attempted home birth records in Canada (Burtch 1987a), along with other studies of modern midwifery practice in Canada and elsewhere. These studies lack the rigour of scientific experimentation (randomization, perfect matching of control samples). On balance, however, they suggest that qualified midwives can practise so as to reduce morbidity, with a minimum of interventions and to the considerable satisfaction of the women attended by them.

The specific apparatus of law in Canada is considered here. The thesis to be examined is that contemporary midwifery practice, whether undertaken by nurses trained in midwifery or by lay midwives, is substantially constrained by current legislation and legal practice. These constraints include the delineation of midwifery as an element of medical practice under the Medical Practitioners Act in British Columbia. This has transformed midwifery from a local practice into an illegal act, thereby effectively transferring power from the midwives and their clients into the professional sphere of physicians and nurses. Other constraints include the powers of discipline and legal redress that physicians can employ against midwives, including the potential charge of practising medicine without a licence. There is also a greater likelihood that police and prosecutors will initiate criminal proceedings against non-medical birth attendants in the event of injury to the mother or child.

Midwives, among others, have objected to the assumption that preserving a monopoly status for doctors and nurses is in the public interest. A growing body of research is available in support of the argument that midwifery attendance is safe and appealing to parturient women. This finding is not fully established, owing partly to methodological problems in the existing literature. Nevertheless, if midwifery attendance appears comparable to or superior to obstetrical attendance, the question remains: why is midwifery excluded or marginalized while the profession of medicine is fostered? Legal barriers to midwifery practice support the professional interests of organized medicine, and at the same time contain more radical, feminist initiatives, including the questioning of power within a patriarchial medical system (Eisenstein 1981, 220). The movement to recognize midwives is not wholly a radical feminist initiative. It does, however, stem from the feminist critique of patriarchy in law and health care. Radical associations have been formed – for example, the Association of Radical Midwives. Other groups in England include the National Childbirth Trust and the Association for Improvements in the Maternity Services (Flint 1986, 238–40). The containment of midwives is sought not only through criminal prosecution or prosecution for the illegal practice of medicine, but more broadly through the power of legal ideology. Considerable power is invested in expert medical testimony, and in the expert application of due process principles in legal proceedings involving midwives. These beliefs tend to reproduce a trust in medical and nursing authority and in legal institutions, with midwives walking an uphill grade in seeking full recognition of their profession. The status of medical knowledge as the lodestar of birth management is to a large extent a result of the consolidation of occupational interests in prestige, income, control of patients, and considerable freedom from state or public scrutiny of professional practices. The central problem investigated in this study is illustrated through a specific instance of "statism." Statism is defined as the transfer of activities from particular organizations in civil society to state regulation (Asher 1981,

43–56). Miliband (1973, 1) speaks of the "vast inflation" of the power and activities of the state such that "more than ever before men now live in the shadow of the state."

Studies of statism highlight ways in which the ordinary activities of people are scrutinized, monitored, and sanctioned through the modern state. Panitch (1979, 10) illustrates this expanded role of the state through the subsidization of political parties' expenditures and influences on trade union activities. There is also a growing literature that is critical of the "commodification" of women's reproductive powers, and the profit orientation of many interest groups allied with birth supplies and technologies (Cox 1991; Mitford 1992).

In chapter two I argue that structuralist theorists of the state offer an incomplete framework in assessing the controls faced by midwives. Structuralist theories fail to take into account instances of sustained resistance to state control of social action. Structuralists question the separation between state agencies and non-state organizations favoured by Miliband, substituting a broader definition of the state. This connects formal state structures (the judiciary, the civil service, the police, the military) with ideological structures: political parties, the churches, trade unions, and specific interest groups, including the medical profession and related bodies (see Poulantzas 1978). The structuralist approach allows for distinct lines of authority between the professions, rival occupations, and state officials, as well as competing objectives among them. The initial encroachment of the state in permitting a monopoly status to medical practitioners in nineteenth-century Canada was largely instrumentalist (serving the interests of members of a dominant class). It was also tied to patriarchical ideology, and excluded, where possible, non-professionals (invariably women) from birth attendance. It has been established that the monopoly status of doctors in pioneer Canada was enforced "in the breach" in regions where doctors did not practise. In such cases, lay midwives were allowed to practise until medical and nursing personnel were present (Biggs 1983; Sigerist 1944).

The contemporary focus of this book, while linked with this instrumentalist framework, will address the complexity and vagaries of state enactments and occupational action through a critical framework, using insights from postmodernism, feminism, and the play of class forces best associated with neo-Marxism. A key point here is that structures of knowledge, once rooted in a specialist cadre and seemingly taken for granted, are increasingly subjected to new evidence, new ways of developing or even imagining legal rights, health care, and women's identities. To the extent that postmodernism has an "affirmative" character, new ways of thinking and action are applied to such profound issues as human rights, peace, and sexual orientation: "The affirmative post-modernists encompass a more optimistic spirit than the skeptics, and they support a range of new political movements ... They encompass 'communities of resistance,' poor people's movements, and therapy groups. They bring together the oppressed, the mentally ill, citizens with disabilities, the homeless, and the generally disadvantaged" (Rosenau 1992, 144; see also Baum, 1990; Young 1990). Borrowing from Marxism, the contemporary state is not simply an instrument of a particular class or set of classes, nor is it a determined set of objective relations. Rather, the state maintains a degree of autonomy in initiating legal reforms and constraining the actions of dominant, privileged groupings. This feature, it is argued, reflects in part the vitality of struggles "from below." It is particularly important to incorporate a feminist critique of patriarchy – within the formal state apparatus, and within everyday cultural practices and beliefs in health care – in understanding the anomalous status of Canadian midwives and attempts elsewhere to limit midwives' autonomy in health care. Attention is also directed to initiatives by state personnel that influence reforms in social justice and changes in criminal justice policies (Ratner, McMullan, and Burtch 1987). The legal apparatus within the Canadian state is assessed in terms of its contradictions, including the tension between democratic freedoms and extensive state regulation of human interests.

The medicalization of maternal and child care is a process against which a number of related issues can be assessed. These include the nature of accommodation to, or resistance against, state regulation. Resistance and accommodation are evident in the occupations of obstetrical nursing and community midwifery in British Columbia and elsewhere. Both occupations seem to manifest degrees of accommodation. Obstetrical nursing has become more allied with medical practitioners as nurse-midwives have sought to be part of a functioning team. Community midwives seek an arm's-length relationship in their involvement with physicians and nurses. Community midwives in this sense challenge the hegemonic status of medical personnel in women's health care. There is some evidence that community midwifery practice is characterized by lower rates of interventions – episiotomies, medication, forceps deliveries, and electronic monitoring of labour – than hospital-based practice. This differentiation is linked with structural pressures on nurse-midwives to defer to physicians during labour and delivery procedures, to utilize hospital equipment and personnel, and the like. This is in turn linked with women's status and the state, especially the concept of patriarchy – the historical exclusion of women from participation in public life, the barring of women from medical education (Strong-Boag 1979, 109–29; Backhouse 1991), and the gradual dichotomy of authority established between men (as doctors) and women (as patients or nurses), both subject to medical authority (Lorber 1975).

This study of midwifery in Canada addresses the contemporary debate on childbirth attendance and its regulation in a number of ways. Published studies of the history of midwifery and the advent of obstetrics are reviewed to place contemporary midwifery in a historical context (Anisef and Basson 1979; Bohme 1984). An empirical study of the practice of midwives in hospital programs and community midwives in British Columbia and Ontario is used to examine patterns of practice and legal intervention for midwives. The empirical study of home births and midwifery practice is divided into three parts. The first is a comprehensive documentary analysis of birth records and charts pertaining to attempted home births with community midwives. The researcher asked community midwives if they had compiled birth records or charts or had access to them. The researcher then requested access to these records to compare outcomes of midwifery attendance with obstetrical outcomes in British Columbia. This documentary analysis provides original data on various aspects of birth attendance and birth outcomes in the province. These findings are linked with other studies of birth attendance in Canada (for example, Benoit 1991; Tyson 1989). This study of attempted home births supports the finding of reduced morbidity for mothers and infants attended by midwives. It also explores how midwifery practice can empower pregnant women, families, and health-care practitioners.

Published accounts of a midwifery demonstration project at the Old Grace Hospital and the New Grace Hospital in Vancouver between 1981 and 1984 are also considered. In conjunction with physicians, four nurse-midwives provided prenatal care, attendance at labour, and postnatal care for 61 women (see Carty et al., 1984). The Grace project has not been developed as an entrenched service. My understanding is that, on average, ten women give birth under the auspices of the project every month. Some midwives view the service as providing an important service to too few women. And some would argue that midwives ought not to use waiting lists, or be unable to attend a wider clientele. In 1991, the Grace midwifery project was temporarily suspended when midwives active in the service became dissatisfied with artificial limitations on their work, including restrictions on the number of women served.

These two documentary analyses are combined with the information gleaned from in-depth interviews with samples of practising nurse-midwives and community midwives, as well as with other people concerned with maternity and infant care and pertinent legislation (defence attorneys and prosecutors, educators, and consumer advocates). These interviews provide a forum for midwives to speak about their work and about the future of midwifery.

Medical and nursing terminology is consolidated in the glossary. Reference is made throughout the book to specific research reports, such as articles on caesarean section rates, studies of induction procedures and episiotomies, electronic fetal monitoring, and evaluation studies of nurse-midwifery and community midwifery (Placek and Taffel 1980; Brendsel et al., 1979; Student Nurses Association 1979; Shenker et al., 1975). Reference was also made to standard medical and midwifery dictionaries and textbooks (da Cruz 1969; Myles 1975).

The results of the sociological approach – documentary analyses, interview data, and state theories – are interpreted in conjunction with research reports by nurses, physicians, midwives, and health-care researchers. The original research and the available literature are used to discuss how particular groups develop accounts of society and their contributions to a given society. I will examine contradictions in formal regulations of birth attendants and the role of the judiciary in rationalizing and sometimes rejecting legal actions (Cotterrell 1984, ch. 7; Burtch 1992, 124–9).

The study of the implications of legal prohibition begins with a consideration of the historical precursor to modern campaigns against midwives, the persecution of midwives in North America and Europe. It is then extended into a review of recent case law dealing with prosecution of midwives under the relevant legislation in British Columbia and other Canadian provinces.

It is expected that state suppression of midwifery, and current efforts to regulate the practice of midwifery, will illustrate features of the way in which structured patterns of authority and domination are mediated through the state apparatus in capitalist society. At the same time, it reveals the pressures for alternative approaches to childbirth and women's occupational freedom, the limited impact of those pressures on legislative enactments and professional policies (such as those concerning birthing practices), and the attempts of the state to contain those pressures through legal repression and ideological persuasion. The theoretical framework in which the above assumptions are explored involves the role of the state as "relatively autonomous" of specific economic or other interest groups, such as organized medicine, and as responsive to countervailing pressures yet integral in the promotion of dominant interests as a whole.

The debate over midwifery practice in British Columbia and other Canadian jurisdictions can be identified as a fundamental dispute about the desirability of granting midwives independent legal status as birth attendants. This debate highlights the contradiction between (1) the ostensible "general interest" served by professional birth attendance, and (2) the radical tenet that legal regulation primarily serves dominant class interests while undermining women's rights to self-determination as mothers and as birth attendants. Specifically, the outlawing or marginalization of lay midwives as well as the subordinate status of certified nurse-midwives in the United States reflects a consolidation of professional occupational interest that is largely intact despite challenges to its hegemonic status (Starr 1983) This consolidation of interest is made possible through legal sanctions that may be directed toward birth attendants "poaching" on the medical monopoly: first, through civil actions against midwives; and second, through criminal prosecution of midwives in the event of injury or death to mothers or newborns (while criminal prosecution is largely eschewed in instances of injury or death occurring in hospital-situated, professionally attended births). There is a precedent in British Columbia in which a person attending a birth was convicted of practising midwifery without a licence (see chapter five).

The legal encumbrances on independent midwifery practice have been interpreted as protecting citizens from incompetent or dangerous birth attendants, and as a way of maintaining professional self-determination, status, and income. The British Columbia College of Physicians and Surgeons has the statutory power to register doctors for the practice of medicine and to restrict the practice of medicine and midwifery by other birth attendants. An exception to this general rule involves outpost nurses working in areas that have few or no doctors – the Northwest Territories, the Yukon, and remote areas in the province. Accordingly, the dominant method of birth attendance is for labour, delivery, and immediate post-delivery to be supervised by doctors, usually with the assistance of obstetrical nurses in maternity wings or maternity hospitals. Even where midwifery implementation is considered, it is often seen as requiring physician supervision in assessments of pregnant women and management of labour and delivery. For those advocating the medical model, it is unthinkable that midwives could be at the centre of things, and call in other expert assistance as needed.

There are nevertheless a number of problems with what appears to be a clear prohibition of midwifery practice. First, the definition of midwifery has not been clearly set out in law. Second, despite potential legal sanctions, up to 100 lay midwives attended births in British Columbia in 1980 (Schroeder 1980). There have been recommendations that the role of the certified nurse-midwife be expanded with respect to hospital-situated births (Registered Nurses Association of BC 1979). Third, there is a contradictory phenomenon of growing support for midwifery training, licensing, and practice on the one hand, and structural changes in obstetrical practice that seek to eliminate midwifery or to "medicalize" it on the other (Illich 1977; Crawford 1980). Fourth, the historical development of midwifery, the imposition of legal obligations to register births through provincial vital statistics acts, and the advent of physician-dominated childbirth in Canada are not understandable through direct reference to case law and statute law alone.

The legal status of midwifery in British Columbia is a critical feature of the growth and contraction of midwifery services. Attempts to prosecute midwives for criminal negligence, a crime with serious consequences for those convicted, including a possible life sentence for criminal negligence causing death (see Bourque 1980), have occurred in British Columbia and Nova Scotia. Legal interventions appear at two other levels: first, the ordering of coroner's inquests and hearings into midwife-assisted births, and, second, the continuing lobbying for legal recognition of practising midwives. Certainly, physicians and nurses are not strangers to the legal arena; however, they are usually faced with civil actions (by plaintiffs seeking damages for injuries, for example), but rarely with criminal prosecution.

The nature of midwifery practice is tied to legal regulation or prohibition in many North American jurisdictions. The abstract protections of law often founder when we consider how laws can be disabling for individuals, or how laws enable state authority (Ericson and Baranek 1982; Burtch 1992, 185). Arguments against legalizing midwifery almost always rest on the premise that midwifery practice is riskier than physician-supervised deliveries. Several research studies challenge this premise (Haire 1981; Levy et al. 1971; Scupholme 1982; Stewart and Clark 1982). These demonstration projects are bolstered by longer-term midwifery services such as the Frontier Nursing Service in Kentucky (Edwards and Waldorf 1984, 10–12). In chapter four, evidence is presented that skilled midwives can *lower* rates of maternal morbidity and of operative delivery (anaesthesia, analgesia, forceps delivery, vacuum extraction, and caesarean section).

This book considers how the midwifery movement emerges and is sustained. Information is presented on patterns of recruitment and apprenticeship by lay midwives and nurse-midwives, on the practice of midwifery itself, on why midwives may discontinue practice indefinitely or temporarily, and on midwives' reflections on the optimal place of midwifery alongside obstetrical care. This information ties in with studies addressing women and the workforce (Marieskind 1980; Wilson 1986; Benoit 1988, 1991). This focus on women as workers is useful inasmuch as midwifery is overwhelmingly a female occupation. It is only recently that men have been admitted to midwifery training in Britain, for example. Considering the near-segregation of work along gender lines historically, it is not surprising that in 1979 only 4 of the 24,000 midwives in Britain were men (Plommer 1979). While there has been some increase in the number of male midwives practising in the United Kingdom, the profession remains essentially female (Lewis 1991). The nursing profession, also essentially a female occupation in many countries, continues to wrestle with its proper role in the hierarchy of health care. Having outlined many structural difficulties faced by nurses today, Salvage (1986, 84) sees something of a sea change occurring within nursing: "Many nurses believe that the old-style hierarchy no longer meets the needs of nurses or patients. It is acknowledged that patients want and should be able to participate in planning and carrying out their care and treatment ... with growing pressure from consumer groups and individuals, the health care professionals are having to rethink their old assumptions about being in charge and telling the patients what is best for him or her."

The theoretical linkage with work and occupations depends upon an understanding of the modern state. The assumption here is that historical and contemporary conflicts among birth attendants, as well as conflicts between these attendants and state authorities, are best understood with reference to the movement of the state into this aspect of health care. By taking criminal action against lay midwives, by transferring licensing powers to medical and nursing colleges, the state reinforces the dominance of medical attendance at birth while discouraging the growth of a more pluralistic birthing system.

THE STATE AND HEALTH CARE

A common problem in sociological research is a tendency toward an empiricism that divorces data from theory (Mills 1959; Menzies

1982, 1). This tendency promotes descriptive research and the pursuit of correlations without extensions into causal relationships among the variables under study. Policy-oriented research has tended toward descriptive and atheoretical analyses, in contrast to the growing critical literature on the state and health care (Twaddle 1982).

This study combines empirical research with a broader theoretical discussion of the contradictory relationship between health care, the state, and the public interest. The literature on state theories dramatizes the limits of pre-eminent liberal-pluralist theories of the state and the politics limiting the rule of law. Critical theories of the state, such as structuralist perspectives, emphasize the play of objective forces autonomously from human agency, and a recognition of the functions served by the state in meeting demands of accumulation of capital and the legitimacy of government and the professions.

A central difficulty with this research is the limited attention given to the state and health care. There have nevertheless been a number of recent articles and books addressing the pivotal role of the capitalist state in containing struggles surrounding health-care services and class, race, and gender (Thunhurst 1982). One major inadequacy in this work is the focus on abstract theorizing at the expense of empirical work on particular instances of state regulation and struggles against such regulation. State theories have also been constrained by a deep-seated reluctance to incorporate feminist perspectives on law.

The intrusion of the state into childbirth attendance is approached from historical and cross-cultural instances. In many countries childbirth was a community event that was later regulated by ecclesiastical authorities (Benedek 1977; Mason 1988, 99). With reference to birthing practices and state regulation in British Columbia, it is argued that the state's designation of birth as a medical matter has promoted a clientele for Canadian medical practitioners by eliminating competing practitioners such as lay midwives. Furthermore, the state's massive expenditures on medical training, hospitals, supplies, medical insurance plans, and so forth has enabled physicians to consolidate their practices and augment their income relative to other wage-earners. Doctors' incomes in Canada have been over three times greater than the average income of other workers since the 1950s (Naylor 1981). A clearer profile of physicians' incomes averaged over time is set out in figure 1.

Government sponsorship of medical services can be linked with a number of social and political interests. There is the importance of establishing a healthy workforce. As well, there are the largely reciprocal interests of the professions and the state in reinforcing patterns

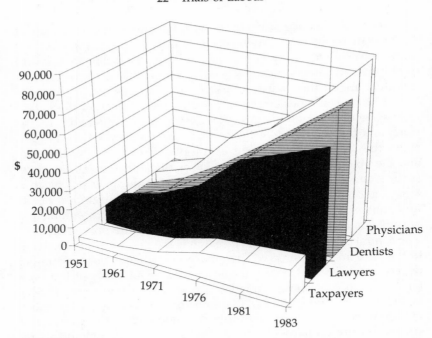

Figure 1
Average Income of Self-Employed Physicians, Dentists, Lawyers, and All Taxpayers in Canada

Source: Taxation Division, Department of National Revenue, Canada, *Taxation Statistics*, annual, various years.

of hierarchy and obedience (Jordan 1987). Some find that the rede-finition of childbirth as a medical matter, dependent on technological interventions, bolsters demands for drugs and obstetrical equipment. Gough (1979, 55) refers to "Marx's own study of the British Factory Acts in the nineteenth century. He demonstrated how the Ten Hours Act and other factory legislation was the result of unremitting struggle by the working class against their exploitation, yet ultimately served the longer-term interests of capital by preventing the over-exploitation and exhaustion of the labour-force." Gough (1979, 62) also refers to the role of the 1906 Schools Act in improving the fitness of the working class (see also Larson 1977).

Social inequality and its near cousin, social injustice, are linked with the production and reproduction of class relations through struggle, including legal struggle (Sumner 1981; Smart 1989, 152–3). The instance of midwifery in Canada appears to reflect self-direction (in decision-making and recommendations) by legal officials (police, judges, prosecutors). This self-direction by officials is less apparent in civil actions under the British Columbia Medical Practitioners Act, such as the charge of practising medicine without a licence. The protected monopoly status of the medical profession is not at issue in such cases, and the court generally has many precedents upholding findings against people practising medicine (or midwifery) without a licence. The self-direction of legal officials becomes more pronounced, however, when criminal law is invoked. This was evident in recent cases whereby the prosecution of lay birth attendants under the Canadian Criminal Code or under criminal statutes in the United States was often unsuccessful, despite representations against the defendants by physicians. The point remains that the Canadian courts have almost invariably upheld the legal monopoly of medical practitioners, including their prerogatives of restricting membership and disciplining members for conduct disapproved by the college.

The theoretical framework centres on the structuralist principle of the relative autonomy of state officials, including legal actors. It is suggested that the Canadian state, including provincial governments, has in modern history become allied with powerful interests, not only in the private sector, but also in the growth of the professions and social services. This alliance is dynamic, and allows for the exercise of discretionary powers by state officials. The midwifery controversy in Canada reflects a general reluctance by many state authorities to engage midwives in their own right; yet, paradoxically, pressure from within Canada and from international sources has led to the legalization of midwifery in Ontario (1991) and Alberta (1992), and to an intention to legalize midwifery in British Columbia (1993).

It is suggested that the medical monopoly over childbirth has been challenged through consumer action and the women's movement in recent decades. These challenges in British Columbia include home births practices of community midwives, the expanded role of nurse-midwives in hospitals, and the acquittal of some non-professional birth attendants on criminal charges; and yet birth attendance as a whole remains largely structured in the interest of medical practitioners.

The autonomy of the state thus appears to be indeed relative to dominant interests. Given the ambit of state control through prohibitions of alternative practice and through enabling actions on the part of the state (billing through the medical services plan, certification for midwifery instruction, and so forth), the role of the state in preserving patterns of occupational dominance is inseparable from the nature of midwifery practice and the legal forces that encumber it. The relative autonomy of the state, as a plausible sequel to what may have been the instrumentalist character of the Canadian state in the nineteenth century, thus implies state recognition of counter-claims along with claims from dominant groupings, as well as state action that intervenes against specific interests of those dominant groupings. This framework may be more applicable to the issue of midwifery regulation than purely instrumentalist explanations of health care or the established literature on professional dominance in health care, which largely restricts analysis to interprofessional conflicts, with limited attention to historical antecedents or larger economic factors (Freidson 1970).

METHODOLOGY

When I first began studying midwifery in the early 1980s, midwifery was essentially illegal from coast to coast, there was little recent case law, and the available literature was very limited. Literature searches helped to establish the general parameters of discussion surrounding midwifery practice and regulation. In-depth interviews using a semi-structured interview frame were conducted with practising midwives in British Columbia. The semi-structured aspect of interviews allows for disagreements and elaborations of general or specific questions culled from the literature review. The interview format allowed probes of respondents' answers; the semi-structured format is suited to an exploratory study, especially since closed formats may artificially limit respondents' answers. Midwives' birth charts and related records (memoranda, correspondence) provided a reference point for inter-views, and allowed a clearer profile of the 1,006 attempted home births in the empirical study. Thus, these research approaches pro-vided original data on midwifery practices and a base of comparison for community midwifery practice with nurse-midwifery practice, as well as contrasts of midwifery practices with conventional obstetrical outcomes of hospital births.

Practising community midwives and nurse-midwives were drawn from a snowball sampling technique. Snowball sampling is especially advantageous for this research. On the one hand, the practice of community midwifery in British Columbia is essentially outlawed, with few midwives advertising their practice. On the other hand, the available roster of registered nurses is not sufficiently sensitive to current practice to isolate currently practising nurse-midwives. Ref-erence to this registry, membership lists of such organizations as the Midwives Association of British Columbia, and adjunctive sources of information served as a safeguard against overly skewed samples that might result from snowball sampling.

Once the two primary samples – community midwives and nurse-midwives – were established, the next step was to contact midwives to request an interview. This was managed through an initial letter that emphasized the importance of the research, assured confidentiality, and provided a brief outline of my interest in midwifery practice and its regulation.

Community midwives from British Columbia and Ontario provided the bulk of birth-related data. Documents from Saskatchewan and Manitoba were included in the analysis of birth records. The sample of practising nurse-midwives was composed of two of the four nurse-midwives active in the Low-Risk Clinic at the Grace Hospital (61 clients between 1981 and 1984), who served as a core group of informants. Reference was then made to other certified nurse-midwives known to those four informants, along with a province-wide register of nursing specialties. The objective was to record features of midwifery practice so as to allow comparisons between midwife groupings and province-wide and nationwide birth statistics. The available documents impose a clear limitation on inferences about midwifery care, or extrapolation to other jurisdictions.

With respect to historical documents, midwifery records are often unavailable, and many are no longer retrievable through oral histories or written accounts (but see Ward 1984). Accurate documentation of contemporary midwifery practices is essential. There are problems associated with the lack of standardized record-keeping among contemporary community midwives, although many variables are usually recorded as part of midwifery documentation. A major difficulty is securing access to records and allocating the time required to code information and to verify or supplement the documentary analysis. Nevertheless, a combination of statistical and non-statistical data was sought in this research. These studies are linked with in-depth interviews with midwives and others, together with reference to much of the world literature on midwifery regulation and practice.

There is considerable danger in going beyond the data in my exploratory study of Canadian midwives, or, for that matter, the available literature on midwifery practice. There have been no scientifically controlled studies on birth practices comparing midwives and other practitioners in North America. Dr. Bernd Wittmann, a medical practitioner and researcher, points to the shortfall in existing studies of home births in Canada: "Data about local home-births have been recently collected, and although to my knowledge the collection has been as optimal as possible, we cannot call this a scientific, randomized prospective study which will stand up to scrutiny. This is one of the problems we face ... for that reason physicians continue to question the safety of home delivery. There are strong statements from all sides that home delivery is considered unsafe, as compared to hospital delivery as it is provided at the present time" (interview transcript, from *Midwifery and the Law* 1991).

Randomized studies are essentially out of the question: women seeking hospital-based attendance for birth will refuse allocation to out-of-hospital midwifery care, and women committed to attempting a home birth are unlikely to accept allocation to hospital settings. The very nature of the birth process would seem to militate against such a randomizing process. Nevertheless, despite the lack of such "pure" scientific studies, there is a considerable body of literature and professional experience that lends weight to the viability of midwifery practice.

The interview schedule also serves to obtain, where possible, documentary data regarding midwifery practice. Missing data were noted. The community midwives providing the records were asked to provide supplementary information where the documents were incomplete. Beyond noting to what degree the records are comparable (between hospital and home attendants, and within both groupings), a key task was to document levels of intervention for overall births. Since there were few births with only one midwife in attendance, the statistical analysis dealt with births rather than outcomes associated with particular attendants.

Additional sources of authority are derived from theoretical accounts of the state. A theoretical review of theories of the state with respect to the dominant ideology of liberal democratic pluralism and competing theories of the capitalist state – structuralism, instrumentalism, capital logic – is crucial to the (more restricted) analysis of nurse-midwifery and lay midwifery in this province. This review will take into account recent observations of a shift toward conservative ideology in Canadian politics, along with the continuing controversy over the functions and legitimacy of the state in advanced capitalist societies. The specific apparatus of legal authority is considered with respect to the regulation of health care and the professions in general.

Research with human subjects is subject to ethical review, with the protection of subjects a primary consideration. This protection was secured in this study through procedures to safeguard the identities of all research subjects. Names were replaced by codes, and the researcher concealed the identities of people contributing to the doctoral research. As noted below, the precarious legal situation of community midwives interviewed by me had to be taken into consideration throughout the research.

Studies of midwifery in Canada are complicated by their legal status. While midwifery is not expressly prohibited in all provincial statutes – for instance, midwifery is not expressly prohibited by law in Nova Scotia – the practice of midwifery is clearly set within the bailiwick of medicine in British Columbia. Section 72 of the British Columbia Medical Practitioners Act stipulates that midwifery can be legally practised only by members in good standing of the College of Physicians and Surgeons. This places a serious responsibility on the researcher. Knowing that community midwives who were interviewed and who supplied birth records were in violation of the act, the researcher took a number of steps to avoid jeopardizing these midwives.

Community midwives interviewed by me were asked to speak in the third person rather than identifying themselves as birth attendants. This precaution was taken in the event that I would be called as a witness to some future legal proceeding. While this was improbable – experts consulted on this matter believed that researchers were not subpoenaed for childbirth-related litigation – the protection of research subjects was paramount. Under the Canada Evidence Act, the researcher-subject relationship is not privileged. Researchers could be ordered to release information for court proceedings. If a researcher refused, a contempt of court order might result in incarceration of the researcher (see Hagan 1984). If subpoenaed, the researcher could testify that no midwife directly identified her practice to him. Therefore, information supplied to the researcher via interviews could be interpreted as hearsay evidence and would likely be inadmissible under Canadian evidentiary rules.

A similar precaution was taken with birth records provided by midwives. The records invariably contained sensitive information concerning the woman seeking midwifery assistance. Details of each person's reproductive history, for example, were carefully safeguarded, and the data presented in this book are presented in the aggregate to protect these women. I asked that these records not be identified as the property of any particular midwife, and that discussion of missing data, clarification, and so forth not be tied to any midwife. The interview tapes, notes, and transcripts were kept in a locked area. Finally, upon completion of the study, the collected tapes were kept in a restricted area.

Some of these precautions, in hindsight, seem unnecessary if not entirely comical. Having people talk in the third person, as if they brought an "imaginary friend" into their lives as children often do, seems to alienate the midwife-respondent. Although it is a technically correct strategy that might shelter the midwife's information or records from a subpoena, this process can demean the midwife and researcher alike. However, over a decade after the 1980 *Midwifery Is a Labour of Love* conference in Vancouver, there seems to be good reason to protect this alegal/illegal profession. Some midwives I spoke with in the mid-1980s have been subject to prosecution (or at least a distinct possibility of prosecution in criminal court for practising medicine/midwifery without a licence). Two community midwives in Vancouver, Gloria LeMay and Mary Sullivan, were convicted of criminal negligence in 1986; their conviction was overturned in 1991, following a successful appeal to the Supreme Court of Canada. Midwives have also been brought into the proceedings of the Office of the Chief Coroner in British Columbia, a costly and uncertain process. Thus, it appears that safeguarding midwives' identities and information was necessary, since a single complaint from a physician, nurse, or unhappy client could subject the midwife to formal proceedings. The 1991 trial and acquittal of an Alberta midwife, Noreen Walker, discussed in chapter five, was prompted by complaints from medical practitioners, not by parents or other midwives.

Another ethical consideration that surfaces during the study is the accuracy of research. Where possible, I recorded data as presented when compiling birth record variables; likewise, excerpts from interviews are presented verbatim or edited lightly to retain the speaker's meaning. Assertions by interview subjects were also critically examined and the comparison of home birth statistics with hospital birth statistics was conducted systematically. As noted above, this was not a randomized controlled study, but one that describes the course of birth and outcomes for attempted home births, and then compares those findings with published accounts of birth interventions and outcomes in Canada. In dealing with community midwives, nurse-midwives, lobbyists, and physicians, I adopted a helpful stance with respect to materials I had access to, sometimes alerting the interviewees about developments in other jurisdictions, pertinent research studies, and so forth.

This research addresses the safety of midwifery attendance, bringing together original data from several Canadian jurisdictions with published studies of birth outcomes in other regions. Proponents of midwifery certification, licensing, and training claim that midwifery attendance can augment conventional attendance by physicians in most births; moreover, in the minority of births that require specialized attendance because of complications, a transfer policy to obstetricians and obstetrical nurses can ensure the safety of mothers and infants.

The evidence from the Canadian experience of midwifery practice, whether in institutions or at home, supports the generally favourable reputation midwives have established in many other countries (see Kitzinger 1988). Practices of nurse-midwives and community midwives have roughly comparable rates of infant mortality, and both groupings appear to have lower rates of obstetrical intervention (for example, caesarean section, forceps delivery, and induction), especially the community midwives. It is important to note, however, that many high-risk pregnancies are managed in hospital. Thus, the home-birth sample may be a healthier sample. This possibility is discussed in chapter four.

This book underscores the complexity of midwives' approaches to childbirth attendance. There are philosophical and policy differences within the midwifery movement (see Benoit 1991), perhaps most dramatically with respect to the viability of out-of-hospital birthing, and also surrounding the community midwife versus nurse-midwife distinction.

The theoretical implications of the study are connected with the longstanding debate over state regulation in general and the regulation of women specifically. Midwifery practice is a crucible in which the freedom of women to give birth as they wish, and of women to work freely as birth attendants, has been historically contained in North America, and continues to be challenged. This study thus explores the nature of the challenge to midwives and their clients – the threat of legal prosecution, barriers to hospital practice and to independent billing under the medical services plan, sanctions against physicians collaborating with community midwives, and possible co-option of nurse-midwives – and pairs this with the kinds of solutions forged by midwives in British Columbia. Two English researchers have identified a "wide variation" in midwives' care for women in labour and in the extent to which midwives contribute to policies affecting their profession (Garcia and Garforth 1991, 45). Concern has also been voiced about the structural limits of time for prenatal care of women in the United Kingdom, and this concern has sometimes been translated into programs, such as the "Know Your Midwife" initiative in London, England (Flint 1986, 1991). For community midwives in Canada and elsewhere, other constraints in services are evident. Midwifery stands as a social movement, one that has attained a higher profile in the 1990s as it has become associated with a challenge to the professions and the laws governing health care.

OVERVIEW: THE POLITICS OF
MIDWIFERY PRACTICE

The following chapters serve to develop the themes identified in this introduction. Chapter 2 presents theoretical approaches in law and the state. The chapter raises the extent to which midwives are faced with rivalries from organized medicine, and to some extent, nursing associations in Canada. The somewhat implacable face of these more established professions is not the only source of opposition to independent midwifery practice. The midwifery debate is thus not simply an expresion of interprofessional conflicts over the management of births. Instead, the manner of state intervention in these conflicts, through legislation and subsidization, is critical in discussions of power in childbirth. State theories are reviewed in chapter two, including critical theories that highlight differentials in economic power, ideological outlooks, and the importance of maintaining social order. The Canadian state is not presented as an instrument of wealthy, privileged interests, but as a structure that has a degree of autonomy in responding to broader interests. This is not to claim that the material basis of the State is unimportant, especially in maintaining patterns of economic inequality between men and women in health care. It is suggested that the more mainstream liberal and conservative approaches to the state, as well as more critical theories following Marxist and socialist precepts, require a clearer appreciation of the politics of gender in health care, and social relations generally.

Chapter 3 brings together historical and cross-cultural documentation to trace the development of midwifery in global perspective. The redefinition of childbirth as the bailiwick of physicians, the relocation of birth in hospital settings, technological advances in monitoring and influencing pregnancy, and the creation of the professional nurse and nurse-midwife are major themes in this chapter. Claims that the incorporation of midwifery into the obstetrical team has been beneficial are questioned, including the assertion that obstetrical techniques (more than diet and hygiene) have dramatically reduced infant and maternal mortality. Another point is the great variation in birthing practices across (and within) cultures, as set against the often monistic premises of obstetrical training (for example, restrictions on delivery positions, length of the second stage of labour, and increases in the rate of caesarean sections). The politics of birth are placed in the context of how women's and infants' lives are jeopardized in some developing countries. Maternal mortality, a rarity in western societies, is far more common in poorer countries where many women give birth without a trained midwife or other health-care worker. This is compounded by poverty and the perils of unsanitary conditions in the woman's immediate environment. The role of international associations, including the International Confederation of Midwives and the World Health Organization, is used to dramatize a worldwide effort to secure safe motherhood.

Historical and cross-cultural perspectives are indispensable to an understanding of the current dynamics of midwifery practice and legal encumbrances on contemporary midwifery initiatives in Canada. In particular, birth as a community concern was recast as a monopoly of doctors – except where their powers were delegated to (outpost) nurses, for instance – and midwifery was redefined as an offence under various medical acts in the provinces and territories. The requirements for proving an offence under such legislation were narrowed, thereby facilitating prosecution for quasi-criminal offences. Moreover, criminal prosecution of Canadian midwives has become more commonplace during the past decade. Just as the movement of the state into civil life is brought forward as a theme in chapter 2, so also has the state become involved in managing child-birth and related struggles.

Chapter 4 presents the major findings from my research on community midwives' practice. A statistical review of 1,006 attempted home births in Canada is contrasted with nurse-midwifery initiatives and earlier studies of home births in the United States and Canada. The findings of the home birth study mesh with earlier findings on the safety of attempted home deliveries relative to hospital deliveries. Rates of caesarean section, episiotomy, induction and augmentation of labour, and perineal tears are lower, sometimes dramatically lower, than hospital outcomes. There is also a substantial diversity in delivery positions adopted by women giving birth at home. The chapter provides an extended discussion of how midwives practise, and of the limitations facing midwives in community-based practices (primarily home births) as well as in hospitals. A common interest expressed by midwives was the importance of trust between the midwife and her client, a trust that was established by continuity of care well before the actual labour and delivery. A community midwife emphasized the psychology of birth as one factor in the delivery process: "The psychology is just not taken into account in the hospitals. A statement, or a change of nurses through a shift change or a coffee break can affect the birth process. A new relief nurse may come in whose energy is totally different. She may not agree with the way the woman is labouring, or may not like 'her' women squatting. In the hospital you are at the mercy of whoever is on that shift, their philosophy and attitudes. In a home birth the midwives have been involved continuously and the birth approach has been worked out previously."

The context of midwifery care is developed through other excerpts from interviews with practising midwives in British Columbia. Birth records are also used to document patterns of practice, particularly the flexibility of midwife-assisted births in allowing different delivery positions for women in labour, while maintaining monitoring of the mother and infant. Tables are used to trace patterns of interventions in home births, contrasted where possible with larger data-sets from British Columbia and Canada. The available information on the clientele of community midwives is also discussed. It appears that this clientele is quite diverse in occupation and birth histories, and is committed to the importance of women's choices in caregivers and where birth ought to take place.

Trials of Labour is not a paean to midwives, however. The praising of contemporary community midwifery often overlooks problems with some practices. There are instances where a midwife misses the birth or is unable to attend simultaneous labours. There is sometimes an "oppositional" ideology that decries heroic, invasive obstetrics while attributing mystical properties to birth, possibly to the detriment of infants and mothers. The material basis for practice is also discussed in the context of an emergent profession (or calling) and the protectionism engendered by the struggle for midwifery. It is also important to note differences among midwives with respect to following guidelines, interactions with clients, and willingness to work toward legalization of midwifery (see Benoit 1991).

A discussion of nurse-midwifery initiatives is also presented in chapter four. Nurse-midwifery appears to be an Americanism, and is somewhat out of step with the traditional role of the midwife as a profession separate from nursing and medicine. In Canada, however, there have been few concerted efforts to establish a distinct role for obstetrical nurses who wish to practise as midwives, with a wider sphere of practice in their hospital-based work. The containment of nurse-midwifery within the hierarchy of doctor-nurse interactions is a central theme in this book. At the same time, the process is dynamic: some midwives with nursing training are aware of the power differences between midwives and doctors, including the reluctance of many professionals to grapple with feminist or other radical approaches to women and birth. A midwife who works in hospital outlined this dilemma in 1985 when she addressed midwifery in her professional role:

I never use the word "independence" in a talk. I always talk about a team, and consultation and collaboration. I don't talk about supervision [of midwives, by doctors] ever, which is how I think they perceive it … I think that physicians are so far behind as a group of individuals [as far as feminism is concerned], perhaps even the women obstetricians. I was very careful not to use feminist terminology or women's issues terminology, because I thought I would turn them off, and that didn't seem to be the right approach. Then, when I heard them speaking, the power and control issues couldn't be separated from the professional, and male/female roles … I use words like "women need to cultivate their strength." I think I left out the word "power," in fact, because I didn't think they could understand that word in a woman's context.

The evidence to date indicates that nurse-midwives are quite capable of managing pregnancy and labour and delivery. In Canada there has been a very limited sphere of practice for midwives or nurse-midwives employed in larger institutions such as hospitals. Most work as obstetrical nurses, providing valuable assistance to mothers, but seldom are permitted to practice independently or to assume responsibility at the time of delivery. Attempts to establish non-hospital settings have not yet succeeded in major centres, and the home has become the key site for independent (community) midwifery practice.

Chapter 5 provides a critical look at the recent history of legal actions concerning midwifery in Canada. One glimmer of hope in this history is the consistent failure to convict midwives for practising medicine without a licence, or for criminal negligence in cases where a baby or mother is harmed in a home birth. More to the point, many legal interventions have provided a stage on which the viability of midwifery has been documented, along with problems associated with medicalized births. It is likely that the weight of scientific evidence favouring midwifery was considered in the decision of provincial governments to legalize midwifery in Ontario (1991) and Alberta (1992). Nevertheless, chapter 5 also points to the costs borne by midwives as defendants in trials, or as key figures in coroners' inquiries and inquests. The general failure to establish a legal footing for midwives seems to be a pivotal factor in the decision of many midwives to discontinue practice. The rewards of midwifery are few, particularly in terms of income; the costs of a single trial or hearing are enormous. This cost is worsened by the tendency to prosecute midwives, an approach rarely applied to doctors or nurses, at least in a criminal context. Chapter 5 isolates examples wherein the uncertain legal status of midwives has been re-examined, particularly in Ontario, where a task force has recommended the implementation of midwifery.

Chapter 6 explores paradoxes in legal regulation and midwifery practice and the future of midwifery. It places the nature of midwifery practice and its regulation and containment by the state in a more critical light. The chapter presents concerns voiced about modern nurse-midwifery and community midwifery practice. These themes include the possibility of co-option of nurses by the medical profession and hospital administration. For community midwives, serious concerns include variations in training and skill, willingness to transport mothers from home to hospital, and levels of prenatal and postnatal care, especially when the mother is transferred to hospital. The theoretical implications of state control over liberties are redeveloped in the context of the data analysis and the recent prosecutions of midwives under criminal and quasi-criminal statutes. Greater attention is given to future research possibilities regarding midwifery practice and to policy development regarding the training, licensing, and discipline of midwives in Canada.

The issue of control is central here: to what extent will midwives be self-determining? To what extent will state forces shape the nature of midwifery practice? The Pavlovian rejection of the midwife as an independent practitioner is still evident, but is increasingly challenged as women become aware of birthing options. Lobbying for autonomy and legal standing continue in the face of longstanding efforts to eliminate the midwife, or to reduce her power as a specialist in birth.

CHAPTER TWO

The State and Health Care

The state is indeed "pervasive in public and private life" and its nature is hard to grasp. But to understand fully the world we live in – much less to contest it – we must certainly grapple with the foundations and complexities of the circumscribing – if not overriding – issue of power.

Murray Knutilla, *State Theories*

INTRODUCTION

The virtual exclusion of independently practising midwives from the Canadian health care system is at the heart of the midwifery debate. In Canada and elsewhere, the considerable law-making and policy-making powers and financial resources of the state make it a pivotal force for midwives. This chapter examines various theories of the state, and offers some links between these theories and the status of Canadian midwives. As a starting-point, it is clear that the displacement of midwives was made possible with the passing of various medical acts and similar legislation in nineteenth- and twentieth-century Canada. The resurgence of midwifery as a modern social movement must again face the nature of the state: the interests it serves, the limits to reforms in state-sponsored services (such as health and welfare), and the treatment of women in health care systems and in law.

Displacement of the midwife in Canada has attracted a number of explanations. For example, those opposed to the reintroduction of midwifery services may argue that birthing women prefer the services of the orthodox professions – nursing and medicine. The provincial acts that govern health services may thus be seen as meeting a public interest in safe health care, with such professions as nursing, medicine, dentistry ensuring a high standard of practice. It has been argued that midwifery, especially as practised out-of-hospital in clinics or at home births, is low-calibre and should not be countenanced by the state. Dr. Hedy Fry, a past president of the British Columbia Medical Assocation, argues in favour of further humanization of hospital births and against home births. Countries that support home birth would thus seem to be bedevilled by this practice, especially since hospital-based deliveries have become the norm in many countries:

I find it sad and a little frightening that the issue of home birth is still a matter for debate in Canada. Surely there is much to learn from the experience of others. In Great Britain, home deliveries declined from 85 per cent in 1927 to less than one per cent in 1984. This drop was the result of the report of a House of Commons committee that was set up to investigate the high infant mortality rates, which recommended that "facilities should be provided to allow for 100-per-cent hospital confinement ... the greatest safety of the mother and child being the prime objective ..." International experience has shown that home births are more risky than hospital births. Women who expose their infants to such danger must be either ignorant, or irresponsible (Fry 1987).

In this approach, the work of community midwives seems to be fused with home births, which are presented as dangerous undertakings. The possibility of birthing clinics as part of a more pluralistic birthing policy is not raised. In any event, a clear message is sent to government representatives and state officials generally: reconsidering midwifery practices that provide a greater range of caregivers and more choices about where to give birth is indeed ignorant or irresponsible. Some argue that even if midwives are safe and desired by a number of expectant mothers, it would be too expensive to implement midwifery training, accreditation, and services. In this light, the midwife becomes a historical curiosity, a predecessor to the more evolved professions in modern maternity and infant care. In this chapter I will provide a critical account of ways in which the nature of laws governing the professions have essentially kept the midwifery movement in check in Canada. The limits to liberal ideology, including the rule of law, are assessed, along with feminist approaches to transforming legal structures so as to strengthen women's choices in birth.

In contrast, there are other explanations of how the Canadian midwife has been moved from the middle to the margin. These explanations concern not only Canadian midwives and their practices, but other jursidictions where the midwife's role has been eroded or threatened and often superseded by medical supervision. This more critical literature points to the established interests of medicine and nursing in governing health care. It also builds on a growing number of evaluation studies that challenge the argument that midwifery per se, or domiciliary midwifery (home births), is riskier than hospital-based birthing. This general approach is not only forward-looking, but also takes into account historical epochs in which mid-wives and other healers were subject to witch-hunts in Europe between the fourteenth and seventeenth centuries. Some point to intolerance of ethnic minorities as a factor in the anti-midwife ideology in nineteenth-century Canada (Buckley 1979, 131–49). Distrust of women's reproductive capabilities and the gradual breakdown of communities of women are also mentioned as influential in the displacement of midwives. Unquestionably, advances in obstetrics worked to reinforce the claims of physicians and nurses that they were the future of maternity and infant care (see Mitchinson 1991).

In this chapter the nature of state policies is brought forward as a decisive factor. Through their powers of law-making and law enforcement, as well as general fiscal policies, the provinces and the federal government were instrumental in promoting birthing care that has been dominated by medical and nursing services. This domination is seen as legitimate, a progressive achievement that stands as the best of all possible worlds in state-sponsored health systems. In Canada, health care is the responsibility of provincial governments. These governments fund and administer many health-related services and create health policies and legislation. In Ontario, for example, medicine and nursing are among the professions governed by the Health Disciplines Act; a number of other health professions are governed by various statutes and regulations. In modern times, the willingness of state officials to enact legislation supportive of midwifery and to plan for the reintroduction of independent midwifery services can make the crucial difference between midwifery that is outlawed and midwifery that is recognized and respected. This chapter places the state as a central figure in the origin of the midwifery debate and in the mediating of contemporary conflicts between community midwives, nurse-midwives, and other health-care workers.

Critical theorists have pointed to the power of law in shaping consciousness and action. There is a growing body of critical literature that regards law as a paradoxical force, ensuring some measure of liberty in western democratic political systems, but also blunting various movements, including the women's movement. Carol Smart, in *Feminism and the Power of Law* (1989), argues forcefully that reliance on legal reforms alone has not served and cannot serve to establish women's claims against male power. "The history of law reforms in the areas of rape, equal pay, [and] domestic violence must surely reveal the failure of law to legitimate women's claims. There are other ways of challenging popular consciousness other than through law, even though law may on occasions provide a catalyst. But it is also mistaken to imply that once legitimized by law, women's claims will not be delegitimated at a later stage" (Smart 1989, 81). Smart adds that the principle that women must govern their reproductive choices is a case in point illustrating how women's rights are weakened through various laws and social policies. The importance of examining results, not rhetoric, is crucial in understanding legal reforms.

The evolution of midwifery as a social movement is analytically inseparable from the manner of government intervention in Canada and other jurisdictions. In all Canadian jurisdictions the provincial and federal governments contribute to the development of maternity and infant care. Medical insurance programs, hospital construction, and medical education constitute major structural changes realized through the state. The monopoly practice accorded provincial colleges of physicians and surgeons is a significant form of power. Prosecutions under the federal Criminal Code underline the extensive state powers that can be brought against birth attendants in the event of damage to women or infants. Not only does the state wield these powers; it also is the site of lobbying efforts by midwives (and other health-care practitioners) to secure a legal status. In short, legitimacy through the state is a central goal for many alternative health-care practitioners, and their success or failure can reveal the manner of state regulation and the interests served by such regulation.

In this chapter, three main concepts will be defined and elaborated. The concept of the state will be drawn out with respect to various theoretical outlooks on state control. The concept of health is directly relevant to the issue of midwifery and childbirth, and is connected with debates over the purposes served by major expenditures in health care. Finally, the concept of justice is important in assessing state regulation of health care, including criminal and quasi-criminal prosecution of birth attendants.

THEORETICAL APPROACHES TO THE STATE

Theoretical work on the state is complex, usually grouped within core political perspectives of conservatism, liberalism, and radicalism, and increasingly with postmodernism (Rosenau 1992). The conservative interpretation of the state will be outlined, followed by liberal and radical contributions to state theory. These theoretical approaches will then be assessed against the phenomenon of midwifery practice and initiatives to legalize midwifery in British Columbia.

Debate over the nature of the state, the manner of its growth, and the implications of state influence on social and economic life illustrates a vital epistemological issue in sociology and in the social sciences generally. This issue centres on the importance of *human agency* and *structural forces* in determining human relations. Social change may be interpreted with an emphasis on how social life is altered through "human agency" (thought, consciousness, will), or, conversely, with an emphasis on the overriding importance of structures – institutions and forces external to the individual – that more often than not shape our existence. This dichotomy – structuralism versus human agency – is clearly oversimplified, and some writers have emphasized the interplay between structural forces and human agency. This interplay is often remarked on with respect to lawmaking and the nature of state policies (Chambliss 1986, 30). Recent scholarly work on the state has tended to feature the interplay between large structural forces (the economy, dominant ideologies, social institutions such as education) and human agency as expressed by individuals, social classes, a variety of associations, and social movements.

For the midwifery movement in Canada, the contradictions of health care, law, and state policies have become very clear in recent years. In this respect, do contradictions in health care require that the state (provincially, federally, and to a lesser extent, municipally) act as a central force to ensure the dominance of particular classes or professions? In this book the state will be interpreted as a crucial force in attempts to preserve domination by privileged groups over other groups in ways that mediate the contradictory mix of forces and interests. State policies are not static, however, or always successful. They may be overtaken by events. For example, in defending the special powerful interests of medicine, hospitals, and nursing, there is a relative autonomy of the state from these interests in liberal democratic states. The fate of midwives hinges in large measure on this degree of autonomy and the pressures brought to bear on state officials.

Many scholars depict the essential character of western democratic states as liberal. The liberal perspective in law, for example, is frequently hailed (and more frequently debunked by critical theorists). Nevertheless, the power of conservative philosophy is also evident in

western democracies – for example, the electoral successes of conservative politicians in a number of western countries, including
Canada, England, and the United States (Taylor 1980). Some point to
the increasing secrecy and centralization of federal powers in the
Canadian state. It has been argued that rather than "developing their
own political capacities," Canadians are increasingly faced with deference to what Woodcock (1990) refers to as "the cult of leadership."
This shift away from a more active, responsive democracy is linked
with autocratic decision-making.

Conservative approaches to the state highlight social order and the
authority vested in the legal order. Order is paramount, for without
social, economic, and political stability, civil life becomes more war-
like, industrial and cultural development is impaired, and life is
jeopardized through domestic and international conflicts. Hobbes
articulated this sense of a common interest in social order that is met
through a strong central authority. Commerce, the arts, the very fibre
of civilization were dependent on a social covenant between individual citizens and the state (Hobbes 1974). In 1652, in *De Cive*,
Hobbes interpreted the state as a public power, a supreme political
authority that was separate from the ruler (the Monarch) and the
public (see Held 1983, 2).

A key issue with respect to state policy is the intolerance of minorities that has often been associated with conservatism. Discrimination
in immigration policy, law enforcement, and work is more likely to
appear under a conservative approach than a liberal state policy
(Gordon 1983). The conservative approach is open to criticism for its
emphasis on tradition and order, even in the absence of convincing
evidence that far-reaching measures and powers are needed. The
abstract value of the "general good" is likewise overemphasized,
appearing often in generalizations about the public or the general
will. Another criticism is the reliance on penalties and force as standard reactions to deviancy.

Contemporary discussion about the capitalist state has been dominated by liberal pluralist principles (Mankoff 1970). Liberal perspectives on the state often involve the concept of pluralism and tolerance.
As societies modernize, some suggest that government policy has
gravitated toward a more positive approach to multiculturalism
through increased immigration and various government enactments
(see Elliott and Fleras 1992, 290–1). It is significant that while liberal
ideology emphasizes multiculturalism and diversity, it does not necessarily follow that racial or ethnic stratification is in fact reduced
under a liberal state regime (Bagnell 1980; Bolaria and Li 1988). For
some liberals this requires a reconciliation between substantive social

inequality and formal guaranteed freedoms. This can take the path of abolishing aristocratic privileges, unchecked bureaucratic discretion, and racial and gender supremacy (patriarchy). Programs to reduce inequality in access to education and legal representation for people charged with crimes are emblematic of the liberal response to inequality.

Liberal-pluralists emphasize the central role of law in making social policies and in the distribution of punishments, rewards, and protections. Part of this legalistic ideology is the importance of the rule of law: that is, equality before the law, procedural fairness, due process procedures, and of course the belief that law is fundamentally legitimate (see Caputo et al. 1989, 3).

There is also an appreciation of spheres not directly controlled by the distributive powers of the state: kinship relations and love are two examples (Walzer 1983). The conservative emphasis on social order and traditional morality is thus leavened through liberalism. Social order is balanced against fundamental freedoms, and the state is entrusted with protecting constitutional freedoms as well as meting out sanctions.

There have been innumerable criticisms of liberal approaches to law and the state. A key criticism is that liberalism rests too heavily on principles and ideals, and misses the *realpolitik* of economics and antagonisms that fuel capitalist democratic societies. A related criticism is that the larger issue of gender, class, and racial oppression is compromised as liberals focus on invididual liberties and rights. In defence of liberalism, some argue that liberals are aware of economics and its influence on democratic politics. Wider struggles for justice and decency are seen as indelibly connected with individual integrity. Michael Walzer argues that each citizen is potentially an active member in the distribution of rewards, penalties, and opportunities: "The citizen respects himself as someone who is able, when his principles demand it, to join in the political struggle, to cooperate and compete in the exercise and pursuit of power. And he also respects himself as someone who is able to resist the violation of his rights, not only in the political sphere but in ... other spheres" (Walzer 1983, 310). Walzer's vision of liberalism is thus not wholly detatched from economics or, for that matter, political corruption. He refers to the "dominance of money" in politics as the most typical expression of power and powerlessness in u.s. society. He adds that primary political campaigns in that country are akin to "commando raids," with citizens largely reduced to spectators (Walzer 1983, 301, 310). The conservative emphasis on public order and discipline is replaced with a clear delineation of private spheres by liberals. The value of these private spheres is consistent with the liberal emphasis on toleration and pluralism. The liberal tradition thus favours limits to sovereignty while protecting various rights of citizens (Held 1983, 2–3).

Marxist theories of the state present a very different portrait of law and social control. For classical Marxists and more contemporary neo-Marxists, the state is the pre-eminent political institution that sustains patterns of class oppression (Miliband 1973, 464). Unlike the conservative theory of the legitimacy of the state or the liberal watchdog function with respect to excessive state powers, Marxist theories invariably recast the necessary powers of the state as forms of domination. The democratic maxim of "the greatest good for the greatest number" in capitalist economic systems disguises how the state serves the interests of the few while claiming to represent the commonwealth. Marxist theories are important with respect to health care, including midwifery attendance, since they incorporate differentials in illness and longevity, along with occupational stratification, in analysing race, gender, and class. Major branches of Marxist and neo-Marxist theory include instrumentalism, structuralism, class conflict, and capital-logic.

Instrumentalist Marxists claim that there is a direct correspondence of economic power and political rule such that the state is linked with a dominant class or set of classes. In a famous passage by Marx and Engels, the executive of the modern state is portrayed as "a committee for managing the common affairs of the whole bourgeoisie" (Marx and Engels 1979, 82). The state may be defined as a system that comprises the government (at federal, provincial, and municipal levels in Canada), the civil service, the military and the police, the judiciary, subcentral governments, and parliamentary assemblies. This formulation by Ralph Miliband (1973, 50–1) builds on the importance of state élites in shaping state policies, and distinguishes the state from the political system as a whole. Empirical studies of instrumentalism thus focus on the class composition of those in state command positions, and also on class-based sanctions by the state.

Instrumentalism has been widely criticized for oversimplifying economic and political developments in capitalist societies. A common criticism is that instrumentalism reduces the relation of state to civil society to actors' intentions, backgrounds, and affinities, thereby limiting the appreciation of structural influences (McMullan and Ratner 1983). This interpretation also fails to account for state interests in controlling the budget and in maintaining legitimacy (for electoral reasons), and the ability of state officials to initiate reforms in the interest of equity and justice. Nevertheless, instrumentalism places an important emphasis on class struggles and the central role of the state apparatus in disguising and managing struggles (Grau 1982; Jessop 1982; Mandel 1987).

Structuralist approaches to the state emphasize the total integration of power and domination in social and political life. Structuralists have also emphasized the play of structures external to the will of individuals. The power secured by physicians through scientific research and clinical practice *and through monopolistic powers of practice under state auspices* poses serious obstacles to others seeking official recognition as health-care workers.

This sense of a social totality that largely determines human action is clearly set out in the work of Nicos Poulantzas. He reconceptualized the state to include schools, trade unions, media, and other (ideological) apparatuses along with formal state (repressive) apparatuses. An abstract, complex structuralist approach was developed in which political struggles are properly to be directed against the state. The state serves as the "factor of cohesion" between various levels in constituting a given social formation. Thus, it is not sufficient to seek to transform civil society or to alter the mode of production without engaging in political struggles against the juridico-political superstructure of the state. The distinction between the private sphere of the family and the public sphere of the state is artificial, according to Poulantzas. His position is that the state assigns the site of the family, and that the family is largely unable to resist or evade this power of the state (Poulantzas 1972; 1978, 66). His approach is opposed to strict economic determinism or historicism, and yet the precise contours of structural determinism are not identified in his writing.

Structuralist-Marxists have been criticized on several grounds. For example, Poulantzas has been faulted for overemphasizing the power of political institutions, and Miliband has commented on the lack of data to develop and ultimately verify structuralist theory (Jessop 1982, 181–91; Miliband 1972, 29). The need to bolster theorizing with careful empirical work has also been recognized by Marxists and their critics. Retrospective "explanations" of economic and political developments and abstract theorizing without reference to a data base are not uncommon. Indeed, some writers point to the frequent clash between "essentialist" Marxist assumptions and the lack of empirical substantiation of those assumptions (Mouzelis 1984; Jankovic 1980, 104). Vincent (1987) credits Marxist theorizing with developing an appreciation of the effects of political economy on human activities, and for its central interest in class dynamics and their relation to the state. He notes, however, that structuralism suffers from several difficulties, among them needless abstractions, and its rather ironic effect of highlighting human agency "while covertly bringing in a new form of super-determinism." For Vincent (1987, 175), structuralism lacks a theory of the state, substituting merely "a negative appraisal of its nature."

Michel Foucault's work, somewhat akin to structuralists' sense of the social totality and the force of objective structure over human agents, differs in important ways from structuralism (Harris and Webb 1987, 58). Foucault writes of the takeover of human consciousness by technologies of control in various sites – the factory, the schools, the military, and prisons. Bodies become "docile," and human action is increasingly monitored, measured, and controlled (Foucault 1977). Foucault's work is especially important in reconceptualizing the joining of power as disciplinary knowledge. These forms of knowledge are convertible into power relations, although the nature of the power/knowledge relationship is complex and not reducible to class relations or economics as such. The "clinical gaze" of medicine (Foucault 1973) is especially pertinent to the midwifery debate. Foucault describes the clinical gaze as an epistemological and perceptual system that builds on categorization and classification of the subject. With the growth of obstetrics as a scientific and clinical operation, powers of observation and treatment became the raison d'être of assessing pregnancy and birth. For Foucault, clinical observation required the joining of the hospital domain and the teaching domain. The family (or community) became secondary to the powers of these unified spheres: "Not long ago the family still formed the natural locus in which truth resided unaltered ... As soon as medical knowledge is defined in terms of frequency, one no longer needs a natural environment; what one now needs is a neutral domain, one that is homogeneous in all its parts and in which comparison is possible." (Foucault 1973, 108).

Such critical theories break important ground in that they recognize how individuals are frequently treated as cases, and how individual choices and perceptions are often submerged within a regimented, disciplinary structure where (professional) knowledge is converted into professional power. Foucault's work has been profoundly important in showing how permeable power can be, and how it is not attached in a predetermined way to a particular class or grouping. Yet at the same time there are concerns about the *sources* of the new disciplinary powers, and thorny questions that are not addressed with respect to law and social policies. Ignatieff expresses some misgivings about accepting Foucault's perspective as is; specifically, care must be taken to consider how state powers, in their myriad forms, can be checked by a democratic tradition. And even the most dramatic forms of state control, such as the prison, continue to attract suspicion and new suggestions about the proper exercise of officialdom (Ignatieff 1985, 94–5). Others have argued that suspicion of state powers is deeply embedded in some political cultures, including Britain and the United States (Vincent 1987, 2).

The English social historian E.P. Thompson concluded that cultural forces can limit the deployment of state powers. Attempts to use the legal apparatus are subject to reversals (for example, jury acquittals) and due process safeguards. Accordingly, while the state may often have the upper hand in dispensing justice and ordering social relations, it is sometimes checked by public pressure and its own doctrine of the rule of law; that is, fairness, natural justice, due process, voting rights, and equality before the law (Caputo et al. 1989, 3). In a classic passage from *Whigs and Hunters*, Thompson warns against dispensing with some safeguards associated with the rule of law: "[T]here is a difference between arbitrary power and the rule of law. We ought to expose the shams and inequities which may be concealed beneath this law. But the rule of law itself, the imposing of effective inhibitions upon power and the defence of the citizen from power's all-inclusive claims, seems to be to be an unqualified human good. To deny or belittle this good is, in this dangerous century when the resources and pretentions of power continue to enlarge, a desperate error of intellectual abstraction ... It is to throw away a whole inheritance of struggle *about* law, and within the forms of law, whose continuity can never be fractured without bringing men and women into immediate danger" (Thompson 1977, 266).

Thompson's writing has been directed against the reduction of human action to mere "vectors of ulterior structural determinations." Thompson has affirmed the viability of historical understanding against the dismissive approaches of Hindness and Hirst, Althusser, and others (Thompson 1977, 1978). His work combines an appreciation of resistance and human agency with a sober assessment of the increasing movement of the state into spheres that were either unregulated or weakly regulated by state authorities. The growth of technological surveillance and intrusive policing policies in Britain, for instance, illustrate this statist movement (Thompson 1983, 479). Another theoretical approach closely allied with the cultural paradigm is the Gramscian outline of human agency. "Human agency" refers to the will and initiative of people, and stands in contrast to the more deterministic theories of the state described above. Gramsci (1971) emphasized human agency in the development of the state and civil society. Ideological and political practices enable a dominant class (or class fraction) to maintain its hegemonic status so that dominated classes and groupings consent to oppression and exploitation (Jessop 1982, 18). Gramsci emphasized the complexities of ideology, class, and law and the potential for countermovements within the state superstructure. Gramsci also encouraged the role of "organic intellectuals" of the political left, skilled workers who would develop social and political policies; they would bridge the gap between intellectuals and manual workers. A synthesis of intellectualism and populism was favoured: "The intellectual's error consists in believing that one can know without understanding and even more without feeling and being impassioned (not only for knowledge in itself but also for the object of knowledge): in other words that the intellectual can be an intellectual (and not a pure pedant) if distinct and separate from the people-nation, that is, without feeling the elementary passions of the people, understanding them and therefore explaining and justifying them in the particular historical situations and connecting them dialectically to the laws of history" (Gramsci 1971, 418).

For Gramsci, then, the potential of social movements was central in an understanding of state domination and strategies for realizing a socialist state. State domination appears as a form of hegemony, the dominance of a "fundamental social group" over other subordinated groups. This dominance is not achieved simply through threat and force: consent is secured ideologically by posing issues on a universal level rather than with reference to powerful groups. As Gramsci indicates, the state is an instrument that serves to shape civil society to the economic structure.

There is also an appreciation of civil society as a source of political change. Even though there has been a statist tendency, the power of the state is limited by the resistance shown by various groupings (Gramsci 1971, 120–5). These forms of resistance bring Gramsci's work directly into the debate between determinism (structure) and free will (human agency), since Gramsci, himself incarcerated as an enemy of the people in Italy, was well aware of the structural forces that limit human action.

Claus Offe has attempted to synthesize instrumentalism, relative autonomy, and structuralism. For Offe, the capitalist state is caught in the contradictions of a capitalist economy. Offe presents the contradiction between the state's interest in preserving accumulation and favouring private appropriation of resources on the one hand, and the requirement that the state present itself as a neutral force operating in the general interest on the other. Just as the state depends on a vital private sector for its revenues, so also does the capitalist state depend on legitimacy of the public. It is important to note that Offe does not agree with the instrumentalist tenet that the state is directly interlocked with capitalist interests. Limits are set on the state by law and by pressures from "strategic groups" such as organized labour (see Held and Kreiger 1983, 487–97).

Difficulties are evident with Marxist and neo-Marxist theories of the state. There is a tendency (perhaps most evident in the Poulantzas-Miliband debate: see Poulantzas 1972) for some writers to resist useful criticisms in developing their particular paradigms. A second difficulty involves the validity of claims. Many of the theoretical works do not include empirical evidence, remaining instead at the level of theorizing. Accordingly, there is no clear methodology for assessing how accurate these claims are, nor is there a clear sense of refining hypotheses or statements (Hagan 1984; Turk 1980).

Marxist-based approaches nonetheless are valuable, bringing forward material considerations as a way of challenging utopian or idealistic discussions of law and liberties. It is important to note that Marxist theory is far from monolithic, with some theorists arguing for a more humanistic or more empirically based appreciation of Marxist theories of law and society. Some see an overlap between the dominant liberal approach to law and Marxist approaches. For example, Bob Fine (1984, 1) recognizes such liberal accomplishments as establishment of civil liberties and the rule of law, yet also draws attention to the "limited democratic character" of law and politics within capitalist societies.

Notwithstanding the parallel discourses within critical theoretical approaches to the state, the articulation of economism (whereby the mode of production shapes specific social and political activities), instrumentalism, structuralism, and culturalism has been useful in developing critical theory about the state. These issues are brought forward in the following section with respect to the nature of state regulation of health and health care.

THE STATE, THE LAW, AND
HEALTH CARE

The instrumentalist approach to health care emphasizes the benefits of state intrusion (statism) into civil society for dominant economic groupings. This benefit is evident in the early legislation in Upper Canada. The Parker Act of 1865 gave physicians a licensing monopoly, including the power to regulate the supply of physicians and qualifications for the practice of medicine. In the twentieth century, with the advent of medical insurance, physicians were guaranteed payment for their services, usually about 90 per cent of the profession's fee schedule (Swartz 1979, 328). Physicians' incomes in the United States are highest (on average) among the professions. Waitzkin (1983, 36–7) associates this financial dominance with a monopoly control that is bolstered through state legislation. Ehrenreich and Ehrenreich (1978, 57) found that the average income of doctors in the United States rose proportionately from about twice the average family income (in the 1920s and 1930s) to approximately four times the average family income.

The economic underpinnings of the relationships between the health-care sector and the state have been developed through Marxian structural analyses. For example, Navarro (1976, 1976a) has developed a theoretical framework in which health services are governed, for the most part, by considerations of political economy at regional, national, and international levels. This means that in capitalist societies such as the United States and Canada, economic factors become critical in shaping the nature of medicine and health. Navarro contends that social relations between physicians and patients reflect a "material basis" that underpins varying degrees of power between patients and physicians (Navarro 1986, 238–9).

The contradiction between patients' needs and profit-orientation in health services is also developed by Waitzkin. He criticizes coronary care units (ccus) in the United States for their expense and inefficiency. The units ostensibly serve the public interest through improved emergency care for people suffering coronary illnesses. Waitzkin contends that ccus generate considerable profits for corporate interests, partly through state subsidies, without demonstrating their value in alleviating the suffering associated with coronary attacks (Waitzkin 1979). A difficulty with this approach, however, is that it dismisses or minimizes authentic contributions to health and other benefits of health-care services (Hart 1982).

Waitzkin (1983) is critical of the misuse of the medical model and the interests served by some aspects of medical technology. He indicates that the development of expensive medical technology and pharmaceutical commodities becomes profitable through state auspices. As health care in the United States has become increasingly commercialized, profits for corporations have been secured. Waitzkin points to a public–private contradiction whereby the state is encouraged to subsidize the growth of private sector health care; for example, by diverting public funds to construction costs of private hospitals.

Waitzkin does not see the state and civil society as a unitary set of apparatuses. He extends Miliband's definition of the state beyond officialdom: "The state comprises the interconnected public institutions that act to preserve the capitalist economic system and the interests of the capitalist class. This definition includes the executive, legislative, and judicial branches of government; the military; and the criminal justice system – all of which hold varying degrees of coercive power. It also encompasses relatively noncoercive institutions within the educational, public welfare, and health-care systems. Through such noncoercive institutions, the state offers services or conveys ideologic messages that legitimate the capitalist system" (Waitzkin 1983, 52).

Others have developed structuralist interpretations of state involvement in health care. Renaud (1978) argues that the capitalist mode of production constrains state solutions to such health-related issues as treatment, occupational health and safety, and environmental concerns. These constraints largely supersede the "volition" of individual health-care workers, public officials, and the population at large. The dominant approach of expertise and health engineering draws together healing and consumption – in other words, promotes a commodity approach to health care. This approach mistakenly treats diseases created by industrial development as natural phenomena. Ischemic heart diseases, various cancers, and mental and nervous disorders are examples of these diseases. This point is raised in Doyal (1981) and developed by Epstein (1979) with respect to carcinogens and co-carcinogens.

Renaud believes that medical knowledge operates within a paradigm of the "specific etiology" of diseases, with analysis centred on the cellular and biochemical diseases of the body. This approach promotes an overemphasis on individual responsibility for health and illness and obscures the structural limitations on health care that are inherent in capitalist societies (Labonte 1983). This alienation of environmental influences, political economy, and health is promoted through the state, the legitimate problem-solver in advanced capitalist societies. The state is cast in Marxian terms as the manager of crises, serving the general interests of capital accumulation and maintaining social harmony while presenting itself as a neutral agent. Thus, government officials are reluctant to address work satisfaction and safety, a reluctance rooted in the commodified relationships of workers to work. Renaud (1978, 115) adds: "[The state] cannot question the basic factor that makes work unhealthy: the fact that workers largely are only commodities utilized for maximum output, efficiency, and profit. It can only act on very limited, discrete, and easily identifiable working conditions." While promoting the interest of professionals with respect to more secure income and increments in earnings, state intervention in the form of hospital and medical insurance programs also serves as a concession to working-class struggles for improved health care (See Swartz, 1979, 335; Morton 1980).

For the midwifery movement and other social movements (see Melucci 1988; Young 1990), the political economy of health care requires a historical perspective on work, law, and health. Doyal (1981) documents the worsened health of the populace in Britain during the transition from feudalism to early capitalism: long hours of work, restrictions on food production due to enclosure, poor sanitation and overcrowded habitats, accidents in factories, and the ubiquitous use of women, children, and men as labourers contributed to a general drop in the standard of health. She concludes that the allopathic perspective on medicine is largely empiricist, disease-oriented, and professionalized. This in turn acts against critical social theory, holistic treatment of illnesses, and the work of "non-professionals." The focus of medical research and practice is on individual pathology and curative medical treatment, dubbed time and again as the doctor-patient relationship. Midwives counter that this relationship is frequently limited in time (short prenatal visits), familiarity, and the freedom of expectant women and their partners to design birth plans. Indeed, women who provide detailed birth plans in some conventional-care settings may become objects of ridicule. A midwife working in a hospital in the 1990s recalled how she spoke up for a couple who had submitted a birth plan for consideration by hospital staff: "They had expectations of no episiotomy, no medications, sufficient time to labour, a chance to walk about. Some staff treated this as a joke. I thought it was a responsible effort by the couple."

Heroic medicine and high-technology approaches to illness coexist, reinforcing the medical sphere. High-technology medicine and the dramatization of medical breakthroughs serve as "window-dressing" and support the existing system (Doyal 1981). Doyal's analysis also emphasizes two imperatives: the production of commodities in the health sector, and the securing of authority relations. Authority relations are divided along lines of race, class, and gender. The importance of gender in health care is central in terms of occupational stratification. The Women's Work Project examined 1970 data gathered from New York City hospitals. They determined that between 75 and 85 per cent of lab technicians, licensed practical nurses, and manual services aides were women; 80 to 90 per cent of workers in the last two categories were non-white (Women's Work Project 1976, 19). The structuring of occupations along gender lines is clear in other reports. In the professional and technical spheres in the United Kingdom, only 12 per cent of medical consultants in the 1970s were women. In 1982–83, 99.8 per cent of nurses in the United Kingdom and 13.7 per cent of physicians were women (Archer and Lloyd 1985, 225). In more recent years, a pattern of more women entering medical school and other professional schools is evident; yet medicine, law, and other professions remain predominantly male (see Brockman 1992).

In their recent analysis of sexual stratification in the Canadian workforce, Phillips and Phillips (1983) reported that two features of the workforce at the turn of the century are still evident: differentials in income (whereby women earn approximately 60 per cent of men's wages, averaged for full-time work) and the concentration of women's paid employment in specific groupings. A recent assessment of women's occupational status in Canada also indicated that women remain concentrated in relatively low-paid jobs (service sector, non-unionized positions). Full-time, female faculty members constitute only 17 per cent of full-time university faculty across Canada (de Wolff 1990, 32).

The segregation of women into occupational groupings in the health and other sectors is linked with market forces. These forces can act in contradictory ways. Fuentes and Ehrenreich (1991) trace numerous examples of exploitation of women in the "global factory" of multinational work. They note, however, that women can organize with respect to pay levels and their work conditions (ibid. 44–6). Another researcher sees waged work in the developing world as providing some opportunities for women, even though such work might reinforce patriarchial elements in the economy: "The expansion of employment opportunities for women in these industries does improve conditions for women in the labor market. In however limited a way, the availability of jobs in multinational and local export factories does allow women to leave the confines of the home, delay marriage and childbearing, increase their incomes and consumption levels, improve mobility, expand individual choice, and exercise personal independence" (Lim 1983, 83). The key to health-care policies, then, is the dialectical relationship between domination and exploitation on the one hand, and changing patterns of health and health services on the other.

LAW AND THE REGULATION OF HEALTH CARE

The specific appartatus of law is a critical factor in promoting and discouraging initiatives in health care. Subsidization of research and formal education are forms of promotion, while restricted access to medical insurance billing numbers and the prosecution of practitioners serve to deter some workers or to limit their practices. Legal mechanisms are a pervasive and decisive force in the restructuring of health care, including maternity and infant care.

As with state theory, theoretical work on the sociology of law is complex and often contradictory. Spitzer (1983) reviews the emerging theories of law that move beyond simple instrumentalism and economism. Structuralism (exemplified by Althusser) and Culturalism (exemplified by E.P. Thompson) are the major competing theories. Both attempt to redefine the nature of relationships between human actors, external structures, and law. A structuralist tenet is that although law is in some sense relatively automous, along with other superstructural features of society, the vectors of legal action are ultimately traced back to the economic system. The reformulation of this structuralist approach by Poulantzas involved a recognition of the role of law as an apparatus that preserves "real rights" of dominated classes (see Spitzer 1983). These rights are embedded within a dominant ideology; consequently, there is an overlap between justice and domination.

E.P. Thompson's emphasis on cultural factors involves an appreciation of the interplay of superstructure and economic infrastructure, as well as a more fundamental critique of the formulation of infrastructure and superstructure. Law is conceived as more than an influence on the material base of society. It is an integral part of the material base (Spitzer 1983, 109).

The relationship between law and the state has thus undergone a contemporary reevaluation among Marxists and neo-Marxists. As Spitzer (1983) indicates, the shortcomings of legal economism and of structuralism have generated a more vital paradigm of law in which law is portrayed as having been created out of an "ideological pool" comprising beliefs and assumptions from all social classes. In turn, the relatively autonomous role of the state – whereby the state is not governed by the will of a dominant class but preserves autonomous powers against direct interests of this class – reflects the contradictory nature of legal ideology and the law as practice: "Legal ideology not only reinforces, enshrines, and legitimates the victories of the capitalist order, it also registers and presages its defeats ... the contradictory nature of law threatens to destroy the symmetry and closure of a Marxism that refuses to acknowledge its mediative and transitory character" (Spitzer 1983, 117).

Other radicals have also been concerned with the hidebound quality of Marxist orthodoxy. Some suggest that modern families can be a site in which progressive interactions can replace patriarchial ones, in which intimacy, cooperation, and child-rearing can exist within a feminist and socialist context (Gordon and Hunter 1977–78, 19).

Eisenstein (1981) portrays the state as an agency that constrains radical alternatives, including radical feminism (see also Navarro 1986, 232). The state is structured such that it cannot allow women's equality with men. The "sexual ghetto" of lower-paid occupations is one instance of sexual stratification that the state, as employer and arbiter of social conflicts, perpetuates. Through law, the state mystifies what women are and what they do. It serves to constrain people's actual options. Yet it can establish "positive rights." Eisenstein recognizes the political power of the state over women while endorsing struggles to secure the recognition of the state. Other writers appreciate the role of "ginger groups" – pressure groups that maintain a critical focus on public policies (Lessing 1986, 15).

In summary, liberalism and conservatism have largely shaped the development of health care practice in Canada. The current interest in cost-containment reflects the waning of liberal programmatic expansion. The state has become a gatekeeper, monitoring expenditures and in recent times implementing cutbacks in services and employment in Canada.

The economic underpinnings of this have been addressed through radical perspectives on the state and economy. Significant disagreements on state theory and political practice emerge between those who view the state critically. The extent to which alternative health care systems can exist alongside traditional ones is a cardinal issue (Mills and Larsen 1986).

In this context, the midwifery movement can be interpreted in the light of critical theory. Midwifery begins with a critique of professional powers, and extends into a critique of media depictions of midwifery, patriarchial elements of law enforcement, and critiques of state allocation of health resources. At its core, midwifery is a celebration of diversity and new possibilities. It not only restores ancient elements of community and female familiarity, but argues for an honouring of these elements. In recent history, the Canadian state seems to have opted more for prosecution than protection of these customs, however. Two examples from England are useful in this context. Dr. Wendy Savage, an obstetrician in London, was suspended from practice in large part because of "her decision not to perform a caesarean in situations where her colleagues would have done so" (Francome 1986). As we shall see with North American midwives, the decision to suspend Dr. Savage provided an opportunity for critics of medicalized birthing procedures to argue for Dr. Savage's reinstatement. It also dramatized variations in caesarean section rates, and raised questions about unnecessary recourse to caesareans and other interventions. The second example involves a researcher and teacher, Marjorie Tew. Tew's research has argued against the equation of hospitalized birth with reductions in maternal and infant mortality. Campbell (1992, 364) notes: "Marjorie Tew's work has continued against a background of great hostility, the non-renewal of her contract by the Department of Community Medicine in the University of Nottingham after the publication of her first paper on the subject being just one example of this. There is probably another book to be written about the response to her work." The point here is that professionals openly supportive of midwifery may pay a price for challenging established practices. At the same time, the movement away from medicalized care and toward continuity of care by midwives is not abating.

Theoretical and empirical studies of midwifery illustrate the nature of state intervention in restructuring health care occupations and suppressing the controversy over alternative maternity care. It will be argued that the state is not a neutral party in the controversy, but that it retains a level of relative autonomy from the contesting parties. A point to be developed in the following section and in subsequent chapters is the importance of appreciating diversity among midwives. They are far from a monolithic bloc: there are some substantial disagreements over the directions their practice ought to take, and the price that may be paid in return for the state's imprimatur of legalization. A related point is the diversity within the state: some jurisdictions have been more receptive to midwives' calls for greater autonomy, while other jurisdictions are so far not concerned with the midwifery movement.

THE MIDWIFERY MOVEMENT
AND THE CANADIAN STATE

Midwifery practice is a complex phenomenon in Canada and other industrialized societies. Legal regulation of birth attendance influences all forms of midwifery, but most dramatically community midwifery. Recent criminal trials have been launched against community midwives, and prosecutions for violations of provincial medical acts have also been undertaken.

Midwives have often received respect from their communities. Whether we look back to the oral histories of twentieth-century midwives in Newfoundland as reported by Benoit (1991), or to texts from eighteenth-century France (Gelis 1991, 109–11), it is clear that midwives were generally treated with respect by those who used

their services. Interestingly, midwives not only served as birth attendants, but were active in other rites of passage: "She brought to birth
and nursed a number of the inhabitants; she also attended to the
laying out of the dead ... By presiding at births and preparing people
for their last journey, the midwife held both ends of the thread of
life" (Gelis 1991, 110). With the advent of medicine and science,
midwives have often been caricatured as witches, harridans, or
simply as meddlesome practitioners (Donnison 1988; Biggar 1972;
Mitchinson 1991). A closer look at contemporary midwives in North
America indicates that they are not so easily stereotyped. Midwives
vary in their experience, professional training, and philosophies of
birthing and politics. A common ground for many midwives, however, is that the practice of midwifery is in many jurisdictions foreign,
and at first glance out of step with what is expected by way of
obstetrical care.

There is considerable common ground for midwives. First, there
seems to be a general agreement among midwives that pregnancy is
not synonymous with illness. Morbid situations will develop, but
birth can generally be managed skilfully and safely without current
levels of obstetrical intervention (often recast as obstetrical interference). Second, it is recognized that the midwife can operate more
autonomously than is currently provided for under provincial law
(which requires the direction of a physician, or his or her delegation
of responsibility where applicable). The dependent status of midwives
is thus generally seen as artificial. This perception is often linked
with the economic interest of physicians in attending births and the
sense of control that some physicians (especially male physicians)
prefer to employ over parturient patients and the nursing staff who
assist doctors in birth management (Buckley 1979).

A third point is that women's right to be informed and to make
decisions about maternity care is vital to the midwifery debate. Midwives place considerable trust in the ability of clients to inform
themselves about some aspects of pregnancy and birth. Midwives
also appear to be less suspicious about women's abilities to give birth
in their own time and way. Fourth, a sense of iatrogenic (physician-
related damage) practice is often expressed. Reliance on such procedures as the lithotomy delivery position, drugs to induce labour or
to relieve pain, lack of continuity of care (throughout the prenatal
period, labour, delivery, and post-partum), and the overarching ideology that birth is a medical event, is seen as contributing to substandard maternity care.

Differences within the movement occur at various points. First,
there is an ongoing debate over the importance of nursing training

as prerequisite to midwifery training. Others favour direct entry into midwifery, or multiple routes of entry, such that nurses and non-nurses could undertake midwifery education. This issue will be discussed in more detail later, but it is one point of disagreement among North American midwives. Some argue that direct or multiple-route entry could incorporate some useful aspects of orthodox nursing curricula, while others maintain that formal criteria are not a necessary condition for midwifery practice.

Second, there has been a movement toward establishing guidelines (or standards) for practice. Most midwives' associations have developed guidelines for practice. These guidelines may require that members do not manage breech presentations or the delivery of twins at home, that women are to be transferred to hospital if their amniotic fluid is discoloured (this may be a sign of fetal distress) or if the fetal heart rate falls or rises sharply, and so forth. A few midwives believe that such contraindications to midwifery management are unnecessary controls on the midwife's judgment. There seems to be some evidence from the American literature that legalization and establishment of guidelines for various aspects of midwifery care may result in more punitive actions against midwives (such as suspensions, fines, or loss of a licence to practise). This is a central paradox of the midwifery movement: in establishing a legal status, which entails the scrutiny and the direct influence of state and professional bodies, are midwives complicit in building their own prison? Some have argued that recent American experiences in states with legal midwifery reveal more frequent and more punitive disciplinary action against midwives than in earlier times when midwifery was either illegal or of undetermined legal status (see DeVries 1985).

Another point of disagreement involves the necessity of midwives working with physicians and the delegation of ultimate responsibility for maternal and infant welfare to physicians. The traditional division of responsibility between nurses and physicians involves the delegation of primary responsibility to the physician (College of Nurses 1983). A counterposition is that midwives can work independently of physicians, at least in cases of uncomplicated deliveries (Van Wagner 1984).

Still another dispute goes to the core of home birth practice. For some midwives, home births attended by community midwives represent an ideal (or near-ideal) method of practising midwifery while respecting the client's needs. It is, in the current lexicon, empowering and respectful of women. Others have expressed concern over the limits of home birth practice. Not only does it dramatically limit the number of women who have access to full midwifery services (even if home birth were fully supported and legalized, it is unlikely that anything near a majority of expectant women in Canada would choose home birth over hospital or clinic birth), but there is evidence that past generations of midwives suffered from some aspects of domiciliary birthing. Cecilia Benoit's (1991) research on Newfoundland and Labrador midwives draws our attention to the bounds of such traditional practice. Midwives' decisions and discretion were limited. The work was often lonely, involving around-the-clock readiness to leave for a birth. Outport midwifery was invariably low-paid, and offered little opportunity for career progress. Benoit suggests that the cottage hospital system was a better organizational structure for midwives than traditional lay midwifery at home. Hospital midwives provided a valuable service, but without necessarily being overworked and isolated and to some extent at the mercy of individual clients. In the modern day, most midwives active in the 1980s have chosen midwifery education and other forms of post-secondary education as a means of acquiring more knowledge and connecting with a wider midwifery community.

My field work on midwifery in British Columbia allows a few observations on the sources of support for community midwives. First, community midwives are able to avail themselves of a variety of resources in conducting their work. There are legal resources available to them, sometimes connected with litigation and sometimes not. A number of lawyers and lobbyists supportive of midwifery remain active today, more than a decade after they first became involved with midwifery and the law. There are legal defences available to midwife-defendants. As demonstrated by attempted criminal prosecutions of Canadian midwives in the 1980s and the unsuccessful charge of practising medicine without a licence (laid against Noreen Walker in Alberta in 1991), these defences have been successfully employed against criminal charges. The various court-situated contests over midwifery and birth-related issues have been accompanied by some political support from opposition parties. In Ontario and British Columbia, for example, the provincial New Democratic parties, through caucus or private member's bills, have supported the legalization of midwifery (Cooke 1984; Stephens 1984). The National Action Committee on the Status of Women also passed a resolution in 1984 in support of the legalization of midwifery in Canada (Sweet 1985). Moreover, the former Liberal government in Ontario was undertaking the legalization of midwifery during its tenure in the late 1980s and early 1990.

A second point is that many practising midwives are aided by the material and emotional support of people close to them – spouses, other midwives, neighbours, family members. Third, resources can be mobilized if a midwife is threatened with legal action. In one instance recounted to me by a Lower Mainland midwife, the threat of prosecution for the unlawful practice of midwifery under the Medical Practitioners Act was not followed through, possibly because as a politicized midwife she was prepared to muster considerable support in defence of community midwifery (Burtch 1987). Fourth, midwives often work in conjunction with sympathetic physicians and other personnel with respect to back-up and transfers of women into hospital. Fifth, midwives utilize various forms of medical technology (oxygen for rescuscitation, sutures for tears) and a variety of communications devices (telephones, answering machines, pagers) in their practices.

Community midwives have also developed the resource of media exposure through letter-writing campaigns to newspapers and contributions to such periodicals as *The Maternal Health News*. Increased income is another resource. Fee increases for birth attendance are especially important in the light of the relatively low incomes generated by community midwifery and the economic strain on family earnings. Midwives' fees for prenatal care, labour and delivery, and postnatal care were approximately $1,200 in 1993. Finally, international support from other midwives' associations and agencies has bolstered the midwifery movement in Canada. The 1993 International Congress of Midwifery, convened in Vancouver, reflects considerable support by ICM representatives for Canadian midwives.

These resources must be placed in a larger context of midwifery containment. Community midwives are liable to quasi-criminal prosecution for the unlawful practice of midwifery, and are occasionally faced with the real possibility of criminal prosecution or proceedings through the office of the chief coroner. Such legal proceedings, along with the considerable media publicity attendant on these proceedings, can have dire consequences for midwives. Ideally, such proceedings might lend strength to midwives' claims that they ought to be respected and recognized as health care specialists. Practically, however, such proceedings can spell the end of independent practice, even if the findings are favourable to the midwife in question. Peter Leask, a Vancouver lawyer who has represented and advised midwives for many years, observes a "chilling effect" created by such proceedings: "[T]he circle of people using that attendant [midwife] or those attendants will spread. Mothers tell potential mothers about their good experience, and you start to get more people – in a small way – taking advantage of this option. Then, we have some sort of either a tragedy, or a tragedy combined with a legal case, and that undoubtedly has a chilling effect. It has a chilling effect on both sides of the relationship. The prospective parents wonder whether it's safe to have babies at home ... Birth attendants who do not make much money from doing [home births], and mostly do it out of a sense of service and obligation, start counting the cost of being caught up in such a tragedy ... some of them say, 'No, the price is too high'" (Peter Leask, transcript from *Midwifery and the Law*).

The personal incomes of midwives are far below those of physicians and those of obstetrical nurses working full-time. Nurse-midwives face constraints in existing law and the policy position of their college and the College of Physicians and Surgeons. Recent initiatives to permit the practice of midwifery on a more autonomous footing required the unpaid involvement of nursing professionals from the Low-Risk Clinic in Vancouver. There has also been a reluctance to acknowledge midwives *as* midwives (since midwifery is seen as a physician's monopoly under current legislation); there has been a recent unsuccessful attempt to define hospital-based, trained midwives as "primary care perinatal nurses." In British Columbia, as of August 1993 there were approximately fifteen community midwives attending home births in the lower mainland area of Vancouver. This is in sharp contrast to a thriving community midwifery practice less than a decade earlier.

CONCLUSION

The practice of midwifery is, for the most part, both constrained by and facilitated through its legal status. A key element in the involvement of the state through its legal powers in what was previously a localized neighbourhood event in North America has been the assumption that midwifery practice is intrinsically more hazardous than physicians' attendance. A related assumption is that midwives require supervision by physicians, although legislation such as the 1902 Midwives' Act in England has established a basis for self-regulation by midwives. A second assumption is that legal constraints on midwives emerge from a public consensus on the appropriateness of restricted birth practices (Howitz and Ussing 1978; Greater Vancouver Regional District 1993).

The constraints on midwifery practice should not, however, overshadow the role of the midwifery and nursing professions in various countries in lobbying for recognition and resources. As set out in the discussion of nurse-midwifery and community midwifery, support has emerged from within the state and within the professions for the implementation of midwifery services. Reconceptualizing midwifery as being governed by the state also requires greater attention to the resources provided through the state. One of the difficulties with the oppositional ideology that appears among some community mid-wives is the bold line drawn between natural childbirth and obstet-rical intervention, between spiritualism and science, and between home and hospital. The machinery of the state can be seen as emerging from popular concerns over safety and welfare, not simply from the logic of capital or the interests of specific professions.

Feminist theorizing on the capitalist state is especially important in considering reproductive issues, including birth. Ursel reviews legislation concerning the role of the state in women's reproduction. She argues that state intervention in Canada "demonstrates both the continuing existence of patriarchy as a regulator of reproduction in industrial capitalism and its change from a familial to a social form" (Ursel 1988, 109). Ursel (1988, 143) also reviews various commissions and legislative enactments, and concludes that the state has not only gained greater control over the supposedly private sphere of family life, but has also restructured patriarchy rather than ending it. This appreciation of patriarchy challenges not only the more complacent liberal and conservative approaches to the state, but also Marxist and other critical theories that do not adequately deal with women's posi-tions in the workforce and their reproductive powers.

The instrumentalist portrait of the state is further qualified by the requirements of due process and procedural rules. A variety of enact-ments, including the Charter of Rights and Freedoms, can be and have been used to offset the potentially absolute powers of the state. The law of evidence and judicial rulings have generally not been helpful in prosecuting community midwives for criminal negligence causing death. Also, despite the hegemonic powers exercised by the state and the professions, the midwifery movement continues a tra-dition of collective self-help and opposition to professional control in health care. The state may attempt to "colonize all forms of exis-tence" (Ewan 1972), but this attempt in law is not wholly successful.

Chapter three provides additional information on the diversity of childbirth practices, including the status of midwives from a global perspective. An important dimension that connects state theory with cross-cultural and historical materials is the need for specificity. Some liberal democracies, such as Canada, have promoted an outlaw status for midwives; other democracies have supported direct entry training of midwives and a broader sphere of practice for trained midwives active in hospitals. The theme of the relative autonomy of the state, evident in clashes within the Canadian courts and legislatures and also evident in this global perspective, captures the structuralists' premise that the state is used to contain initiatives from relatively powerless groups. This containment is nonetheless subject to change, and the sources of change emerge not only in civil society but within the very framework of the state. This is an apt theme in the Canadian context: whereas the monopoly status of medicine in childbirth reflects an instrumentalist perspective, there is evidence that the medical thrall is diminishing in North America as other health professions demand legal status (Starr 1978, 1983; Coburn et al. 1983). Groups that currently enjoy legal status may also mobilize against unwarranted interference in their work. A case in point is recounted by the Association of Radical Midwives (ARM) in England. Although midwives in England have had legal status under the Midwives Act since 1902, there are concerns over limitations imposed on their work. In 1986 ARM published several proposals to restructure maternity services in England. The authors indicate that many midwives are dissatisfied with the fragmented care offered to pregnant women, and that midwives are hardly considered "practitioners in their own right" (Association of Radical Midwives 1986). The agency of midwives is also apparent in the way the argument against the greater empowerment of midwives can be turned on its head. Rather than seeing midwives as duplicating doctors' services in maternity care, the ARM paper places midwives at the centre of such care. This woman-centred approach offsets the possible trap of women moving to alternative birth centres (ABCs) that are not consumer-oriented and -managed, but largely controlled by professional interests: "Much of the obstetric care given by GPs at the moment results in either duplication of or failure to make full use of midwives' skills. We recognize that the GP has a long term commitment to the family and could be the source of much valuable background information in such cases" (Association of Radical Midwives 1986). In the United States, the opposition to home births, and to midwives' taking a more central role in assisting with deliveries and pregnancies generally, has been fierce. And even though the arguments may become less inflammatory and more subtle as midwives and doctors vie for access to birthing women, there is still a depiction of superior caregivers versus their enemies (Treichler 1990, 126–8).

The vast literature on the state serves the useful purpose of speaking to the issue of power and its translation into control over thought and practices. The very hegemony of the medical profession in western countries rests not only in its claims to powers but in its special status as a prestigious profession. Obviously, there are contradictions evident here, not least in the paradox of a self-governing, self-directing profession that is, in some countries such as Canada, dependent on the public education (of doctors) and publicly supported resources such as health insurance plans and the running of hospitals and clinics. Nonetheless, the translation of power into action seems far easier for the medical profession than for ejected groups such as midwives. The strength of occupational monopolies such as medicine includes its ability to manage allied groups in such a way that medical prestige and income are not substantially threatened (Larkin 1983, 4).

These modern conflicts surrounding monopolistic professional powers, safety of infants and mothers, and women's right to choose the place of birth and birth attendants become understandable when two dimensions are considered: the historical dimension of control over childbirth, and the cross-cultural variations in birthing practices, particularly in the role played by midwives. Chapter three elaborates on these points and on the pivotal role of the state in shaping the historical directions and, to some extent, the cross-cultural expressions of midwifery and birth practices. The point to be developed in this book is that the mistrust of midwives in Canada has a long if not very distinguished pedigree. Arguments against midwives have tended to emerge from those professions that have become responsible for assessing and treating diseases: medicine and nursing.

Theories of the state are useful in assessing the politics of resistance to midwifery, including of course groups within nursing and medicine who favour the implementation of midwifery. The role of the state in safeguarding the material interests of the professions has been strong, yet a growing criticism of the limitations of the intervention-oriented medical model has challenged the equation of professional management of birth equalling better outcomes, including women's satisfaction with birthcare. Feminist critiques of the nature of reproductive rituals and technology pose an important challenge to medicalization, and serve to highlight women's choices in reproduction (Cox 1991). Patriarchial control measures in routine obstetrics are thus the subject not of passive acceptance, but oftentimes of questioning. Thus, the hegemonic power of the medical profession in "presiding" over births, as well as the restrictive legislation that provinces have traditionally enacted, face growing criticisms, especially in their outlawing what might be termed more holistic professions, such as midwifery and chiropractic (see Biggs 1988). A combination of structuralist theory, feminist theorizing, and especially the role of human agency in protesting restrictive controls (and presenting innovative approaches in maternity and infant care) highlights the obstacles midwives and their supporters face in overcoming legislative restrictions and the material interests of the more established players in health care.

CHAPTER THREE

Historical and Crosscultural Aspects of Midwifery

Then the king of Egypt said to the Hebrew midwives, one of whom was named Shiph'rah and the other Pu'ah, "When you serve as midwife to the Hebrew women, and see them upon the birthstool, if it is a son you shall kill him; but if it is a daughter, she shall live." But the midwives feared God, and did not do as the king of Egypt commanded them, but let the male children live.

Exodus 1: 15–16

And if there is a single piece of wisdom that has more humanity in it than any other it is this: befriend the womb.

Hugh Hood, *Reservoir Ravine*

INTRODUCTION

Thousands of years separate the biblical account of the midwives' defiance of Herod and the current conflicts over state policies concerning midwifery. This chapter provides an overview of major developments in the evolution of midwifery worldwide. Two broad areas are considered. The first is historical developments in formalized midwifery practice, with special attention to England, continental Europe, the United States, and Canada. This discussion goes beyond Canada's anomalous situation in not recognizing midwifery practice. In Europe, ecclesiastical and state regulation and advances in science and obstetrics profoundly affected traditional birthing cultures. Birth was claimed as part of the medical terrain. In North America, midwives were often subjected to antagonistic campaigns by medical and nursing associations. Historically, deep conflicts and competition emerged between midwives, who had attended births since ancient times, and aspiring male medical practitioners. These conflicts have not spelled the eradication of the midwife, but have foreshadowed ongoing conflicts surrounding the proper practice of midwifery as a health profession.

The diversity of midwife practices in various cultures is explored in the second part of this chapter. In virtually all cultures women have been customarily been responsible for assisting at births. Birth attendance and assistance after birth often involved kin and neighbours. Birth was a local event, unadorned with technological aids or monitoring devices as we know now them. The advent of professionalized midwifery, or the displacement of midwifery by medical and nursing personnel, is set in the wider framework of technological advances, centralization of maternity services, and formal bureaucratic structures. These crosscultural materials are used to argue for the viability of community-based approaches to birthing (Askew et al., 1989; Rifkin 1990), and to document the seriousness of infant and maternal mortality rates in many developing countries (Maine n.d.; Kwast 1991, 1993). The transformation of birth is a complex process, riddled with contradictions and opportunities. Wider structures of medical ideology, opposition to medicalization, and structural limits imposed by customs and by disparities in wealth are also reviewed across several cultures.

HISTORICAL PERSPECTIVES ON MIDWIFERY

The evolution of midwifery in Europe reflects technological advances in the medical sciences and the changing patterns of control through the professions and the influence of the state. These structural changes have contributed to the eclipsing of the traditional midwife by physicians and her near-replacement by the nursing and nurse-midwife professions in North America. This intrusion into what was historically women's sphere transformed the role of women in maternity care. This intrusion means that reproduction is usually mediated and controlled by an élite of primarily male physicians (Oakley 1980, 8–10). This intrusion was contested and limited to an extent by custom and by concerns about the improper takeover of midwifery practice. Nonetheless, the traditional role of the midwife was changed with the growth in number of rival practitioners, and new knowledge concerning anatomy, physiology, and obstetrics.

Bohme (1984) traces four phases in the social history of European midwives. The first phase, solidary aid, is traced to the early days of civilization. Knowledge of childbirth was gained by witnessing births and through personal experience. Giving birth was a necessary aspect of becoming a midwife. Solidary aid was based on the communal involvement of women assisting other women during labour, delivery, and the post-partum period.

The second phase is that of office. The ecclesiastical overseeing of life in the Middle Ages was extended to childbirth. Midwives were appointed and licensed by the church to ensure that the moral character of birth attendants befitted the office. The midwife was not only to provide care to women, but also to thwart abortions, to watch for substitutions (changelings), and to prevent infanticide. Paternity was established by midwives, and newborns were baptized by midwives. Midwives could not profit by their work. The office of midwife sought "poor but honest" practitioners (Bohme 1984, 375).

The third phase, traditional profession, marked the transition from an assigned office to a more secular conflict between midwives and male physicians at the beginning of the eighteenth century. Surgeons and barber-surgeons, once restricted to performing caesarean sections or extracting stillborn babies (or babies who could be removed otherwise), asserted their superiority via innovations such as the forceps and anaesthesia. The exclusion of women from the universities and the development of gynecology and surgery further reduced the province of the appointed midwife (Bohme 1984, 375). The current status of midwifery as a modern profession is the fourth phase discussed by Bohme, in which midwives become self-regulating and licensed, a system that predominates in modern Europe. Specialized training of midwives, the establishment of local and international associations, and the combination of theoretical knowledge and practical midwifery skills exemplify this phase.

The growth of new structures of knowledge surrounding obstetrics and midwifery was influential in shaping the role of midwives. In contrast to its neighbourly quality in earlier times, the phenomena of pregnancy, birth, and post-partum care fell under the mantle of scientific management. This scientific basis revolutionized the management of birth. In some important respects this revolution benefited mothers and infants; in other ways, birthing lore and respect for women's ability to give birth were eroded (Lang 1972). The "miracles" associated with heroic medicine and the less dramatic aspects of the work of medical and nursing disciplines, were not always extended to lay midwives or aspiring midwives.

Descriptions of the historical development of English midwifery are rich, and provide a useful account of a nation that has entrenched midwifery care, but not without criticism of the limits facing many midwives. Jean Donnison (1977, revised 1988) has provided a comprehensive history of English midwives, and documents the rivalries that emerged over maternity and infant care. In *Midwives and Medical Men* (1977) she traces these rivalries, accompanied by the growth of professionalized medicine and nursing. English midwives in the Middle Ages were likely to be middle-aged married women who had given birth. Donnison adds that women were active not only as midwives but in the healing arts more generally. Medicine and surgery were offered by women active in charitable work among the poor, and some women practised medicine for pay. In England, "until the thirteenth century practice in the whole field of medicine appears to have been open to all, men and women, whether possessed of education or training, or not" (Donnison 1977, 2–3).

The customary practice of lay midwifery was altered dramatically with the advent of barber-surgeons' guilds in the thirteenth century. Surgeons were granted an exclusive status in towns and surrounding areas. They were often designated as the appropriate birth attendants for abnormal deliveries. Surgeons were thus permitted to perform instrumental deliveries and deliveries by Caesarean section. Donnison (1977, 2) concludes that guild membership seems to have been open to women, "but their number does not appear to have been large."

Donnison outlines the wide compass of human affairs subject to church control. Episcopal licensing was a form of midwifery regulation that influenced birth attendance. As noted earlier, midwives were to be of good moral character. They could be required to take an oath and to produce witnesses to vouch for their good character. They were obliged to see that babies were christened in accordance with church doctrine. Midwives served also to inquire into fathers' identities in cases of bastardy. Along with these obligations, midwives were forbidden to practise abortions or to be involved in witchcraft (Donnison 1977, 4). The licensing of physicians was vested in church authorities in England in 1511, while the informal regulation of midwives by the church was legalized in 1512. Power over birth attendants, particularly midwives, was thus transferred from the community and the parish and centralized at the bishops' level in the church hierarchy.

Midwives were hindered by church proscriptions on their conduct and by the lack of an internationally recognized knowledge base. The absence of a knowledge base contributed to the limited powers of community midwives in resisting the growth of scientific obstetrics developed in France and adapted in Britain (see Arney 1982, 21–9). Fifteenth-century English midwives were sometimes denounced as agents of the devil, but were not subjected to the inquisitorial punishments to the same degree as midwives in continental Europe (Donnison 1988, 17; Ben-Yehuda 1980).

Midwives in Europe were denounced as witches, and thousands of midwives and female healers were executed. Donnison sees this campaign against heresy as rooted in misogyny. One book, *Malleus Maleficarum* (*The Hammer of Witches*) is described as "a classic in misognynist writing" (Donnison 1988, 17, 40–1). A document written in 1484 by two men active in the Inquisition, the *Malleus Maleficarum* justified the prosecution of midwives and other healers. Donnison (1988) believes that this book and witch-hunting were premised on the belief that women's essence was irrational and "passive," and inferior to men's essence and talents. She notes that the thesis of the *Malleus Maleficarum* "is that women, because of their greater 'carnality,' are easily tempted to serve the Devil, who in this 'twilight' of the world was using them in his attempt to overthrow Christendom" (Donnison 1988, 17).

The witch-hunts endured for centuries, shored up by the power of formal legal procedures. In America, the infamous Salem witch trials of 1692 led to the execution of fourteen women and six men (Williams and Adelman 1992, 200). Ehrenreich and English (1973, 9) criticize interpretations that attribute the witch-hunts to a kind of hysteria; rather, the hunts "were well-organized campaigns, initiated, financed and executed by Church and State." These vilification campaigns were not without their critics. Some opposed the encroachment of male midwives in birth on grounds of modesty as well as the unnatural methodologies and inferior skills of male attendants. In *A Treatise on the Art of Midwifery* (1760), Elizabeth Nihell criticized the lower pay available to women attendants relative to men (Arney 1982, 30–1).

Beginning in 1890, many midwives' bills were proposed in England. The first act governing midwives was passed in 1902. The Midwives Act of 1902 followed the efforts of the Midwives' Institute and its supporters to gain legal recognition and a protected status in law. Midwifery was not given an autonomous status, however. This result followed a longstanding pattern of medical opposition to the registration of midwives. Medical authorities were generally agreeable to registering midwives only if medical control was secured over registration. It appears that general practitioners were especially wary of midwives, who were seen as competitors for family practice. Opposition to midwives also fed on the notion that midwifery would, almost by natural selection, give way to medical care in future. The science of obstetrics, aided by such instruments as the forceps (Nagy

1983–4), heralded the eclipse of the ancient art of midwifery by the medical model: "In the more affluent and educated world of the future, every woman would be delivered by a doctor, and the midwife, a relic of a less civilized past, would vanish from the scene" (Donnison 1977, 158).

The Midwives Act of 1936 subjected the midwives to local authorities. It also provided broader grounds for deregistration on grounds of professional misconduct. The private lives of midwives were open to scrutiny. The Midwives Act enacted in 1936 reflected concerns over the falling birth rate in England and the likelihood of war. Local authorities were to secure salaried, full-time midwifery services adequate to the citizenry. The act also promoted the development of professional midwifery: unqualified midwives were banned from attending birth in any capacity (Donnison 1977, 191). The amended Midwives Act of 1951 stipulated that the board could strike off midwives whose conduct unrelated to their work brought the profession into disrepute (Donnison 1988, 181). Some have suggested that the greater degree of institutionalization of midwifery in Britain (relative to the United States) hinges in part on the lack of regulation of midwifery in colonial America, and the failure to establish midwifery as a centrally controlled institution in the face of opposition by organized medicine (Anisef and Basson 1979).

Clearly, the 1902 Midwives Act was an important achievement for midwifery in the United Kingdom. The act helped to secure midwifery practice in the face of ongoing efforts to eliminate midwifery altogether. It maintained female attendance in childbirth as a feature of English society. Moreover, the scope of "improper practice" was more broadly defined. It was especially important that the medical profession secure "a dominant voice" in midwifery governance (Donnison 1988, 74).

European municipalities gradually devised systems providing for midwifery care and licensing. Donnison believes that while the midwives' character was important for municipal authorities, greater emphasis came to be placed on the midwives' "technical competence." Midwives were examined by other midwives or physicians, and sometimes by a combination of more experienced midwives and physicians, constituting an examining board. These municipal systems helped to establish midwifery practice, but by the same token served to limit its operations. Donnison cites the requirement that midwives seek medical assistance for difficult births, and the prohibition against midwives' using various obstetrical devices to extract infants. In Strasbourg, for example, midwives who used sharp objects (hooks) to extract infants could be subject to the death penalty (Donnison 1977, 174–5).

A key point is that these early regulations were directed toward the exclusive practice of some forms of midwifery, an approach that carried penalties for those violating regulations. This produced "a system of licensing skilled and approved practitioners, and for the punishment and suppression of the rest" (Donnison 1977). There were of course exceptions in the enforcement of regulations. Midwives who could not afford the licensing fee might continue to practice, with authorities turning a blind eye if they practised among the needy (Donnison 1977).

The declining prestige of midwives throughout Europe is traced to several factors. Scientific advances beginning in the sixteenth century were undertaken by men. As labour and delivery became the focus of science and medicine, "operative midwifery" became more commonplace, spreading from France throughout Europe (Donnison 1977, 10–11). Donnison concedes that some midwifery practices at this time posed dangers to mothers and infants. She adds two important points: first, that midwives were not alone in engaging in unjustifiable practices, and, second, that there was no provision at this time "to help midwives improve their professional competence" (Donnison 1977, 11).

For Donnison (1988, 34) from 1720 onwards, midwives were "losing ground" to men. The ancient art was depicted as an anachronism, in contrast to science and medicine. Male practitioners not only established their power in managing abnormal births; they also began to attend ordinary births in greater numbers. Donnison notes men's advantages in gaining formal instruction in obstetrics, as well as the critical power of using forceps to assist in deliveries. The forceps could be life-saving for mothers and infants, and midwives had customarily done without such devices (Donnison 1988, 12). Men's involvement in births intensified, despite opposition from midwives and dissent from some doctors. Opponents voiced concerns about female modesty, as well as principled objections to the exclusion of midwives from new knowledge. John Douglas, a London surgeon, argued in his *Short Account of the State of Midwifery in London, Westminster &c* (1736) that it would be better to provide instruction for midwives rather than admonishing them for their lack of skills (see Donnison 1977, 23–24).

Donnison's work is remarkable for its detailed account of the allies and critics of midwives. Some innovations, such as the creation of lying-in hospitals in Dublin, London, and other cities beginning in the late eighteenth century, offered instruction opportunities to female students. Overall, however, the creation of a class of trained midwives was frequently blocked by limited opportunities and cat-calls from their medical competitors: "[Male practitioners] exagger-ated the dangers of childbirth and frightened women into believing that extraordinary measures, and therefore male attendance, were more generally necessary than they actually were. At the same time they made the most of every occasion to denigrate the understanding and competence of midwives, and to blame them, however unjustly, for anything that went wrong" (Donnison 1977, 29).

Donnison notes that for 250 years midwives had been subject to encroachments on their practice, with very little improved training and few opportunities for practice. Midwives lacked their own schol-arly journals, midwifery textbooks, professional societies, and, above all, political organization and alliances. Midwives were not com-pletely without support from outside the ranks of midwifery. Florence Nightingale, for example, not only promoted nursing as a vocation, but also favoured the establishment of government-sponsored schools of midwifery. The women's movement in England was also active in support of midwives and women who were barred from entering medical schools. Even as midwifery and improvements to women's legal, social, and occupational status were promoted, Don-nison (1988, 92–3) concludes that midwives continued to lose ground to other caregivers.

The Female Medical Society (1862–1872) was an important force in the midwifery movement in England. Although it lasted only a decade, and did not produce a large number of qualified midwives, Donnison credits this society and its supporters with strengthening the argument for midwifery. The society, led by Dr. James Edmunds, joined with wider movements of the day in seeking improvements in public health (including temperance and the prevention of conta-gious diseases), and argued publicly in favour of midwifery practice. The lack of adequate midwifery attendance for mothers and infants and the artificial obstructions to talented women seeking to practice midwifery were decried by the society (see Donnison 1977, 73–4).

In Germany, concerns were expressed about unregulated mid-wifery practices. These concerns included illiteracy and superstition among midwives, along with injuries to women (caused by the prac-tice of manually removing the placenta) and to infants resulting from incorrect cutting of the infant's frenum (the small ligament controlling the movement of the tongue: see Shorter 1982). These concerns led to formal regulations specifying the responsibilities of midwives and physicians in Germany. One requirement of late fifteenth-century and early sixteenth-century urban ordinances in Germany was that midwives were required to summon physicians for advice or direct assistance in complicated deliveries (Benedek 1977). More brutal measures were also taken against midwives. Witch-hunting resulted in the executions of thousands of midwives, and it appears that those not affiliated with a man were especially vulnerable to witch hunts (Midelfort 1972; Daly 1978, 184–5). In spite of this inquisitional legacy, midwifery found its foothold in Europe as midwifery schools became established in the eighteenth century (Donnison 1977, 40).

The opposition to lay midwives was evident in France. As Theophile Roussel indicated in 1874, many birth practices of the day were seen as unenlightened. In eighteenth century France, child care given by "wet" and "dry" nurses not uncommonly resulted in infant deaths through neglect (Badinter 1979; Colette 1979, 128). The menace of untrained midwives was denounced: "Notwithstanding the disinterested counsel of physicians and enlightened persons, the force of habit, the brutish stubborness of the peasants, and the foolish advice of the midwives maintain practices that are fatal to children whose health needs are poorly attended to" (cited in Donzelot 1979, 30–1).

The French government also established midwifery instruction at the Hôtel Dieu Hospital in Paris. Midwives received instruction in midwifery, textbooks on midwifery were made available, and lying-in hospitals were established (Donnison 1977, 40). Donnison concludes that government intervention was to the benefit of French and German midwives. That said, by the late nineteenth century midwives in France "were gradually being brought under the authority of the medical profession," while in Germany midwives were increasingly relegated to attending "routine" births, and men became more prominent in attending wealthier women (Donnison 1977, 85).

The situation was worsening in England. Government-subsidized instruction was lacking in the eighteenth century, and charitable institutions were not greatly involved in furthering midwifery practice. By the 1720s male midwives were becoming more prominent in attending normal and abnormal deliveries (see Donnison 1977, 21). Without adequate financial rewards for the practice of midwifery, it seemed inevitable that midwives in England were destined to disappear altogether as men became more and more involved in managing births. Donnison notes that the practices of male midwives became more pervasive in England than in any other European country.

The growth of state authority served to mediate the growing rivalry between traditional female midwives and the male midwives who aspired to attend a greater proportion of births. Midwives and medical practitioners were vilified and satirized, and appeals were made to government for recognition of the superior skills of either profession. Competition between midwives and medical practitioners is still very much in evidence in western obstetrics: midwifery, as a profession independent of nursing and medicine, continues to face opposition on many fronts (Picard 1991).

Midwifery in Canada

There is an underside to every age about which history does not often speak, because history is written from the records left by the privileged. We learn about politics from the political leaders, about economics from the entrepreneurs, about slavery from the plantation owners, about the thinking of an age from its intellectual élite.

Howard Zinn, *The Politics of History*

The historical study of midwifery in Canada has until recently suffered from the elitist view outlined by Zinn. Historical approaches have favoured a version of history written "from above," not from a working-class perspective (Shortt 1981). Biographical accounts of eminent physicians and chronicles of dramatic medical advances are featured in this antiquarian approach, while accounts by working-class people are absent or minimal. Nellie McClung (1935) stated that those who did "the work of the world" were not written about by historians. There is, however, a renewed interest in social history, and in the use of oral histories (Thompson 1978) to explore events and experiences ignored in existing accounts. Women's experiences have often been "hidden from history" (Rowbotham 1973). Several Canadian historians have recovered some of these histories (see, for example, Strong-Boag 1988; Backhouse 1991; Creese and Strong-Boag 1992), including accounts of the ways in which women's reproduction was regulated (McLaren and McLaren 1986; Mitchinson 1991).

The absence of historical documentation by and about Canadian midwives is most evident in the lack of records and documents of lay midwives in frontier and post-frontier eras. Lay midwives in Canada rarely kept systematic records. For example, documentation on births attended by a Regina-based midwife between 1916 and 1918 noted only the date, the name of the mother, whether a doctor was present, and the street address ("Mrs. F.A. Wayling"; see also the records of Jane Hamilton Sorley, 1851–1893, "Five Islands, N.S., Midwife"). Mrs. Sorley's records contained only the date of the child's birth and the mother's name. Records from Ukrainian, Scandinavian, Acadian, and Quebecoise midwives do not appear to have been translated into English (but see Ward 1984). The absence of written records has also been observed in historical accounts of lay midwifery in the United States (Donegan 1978, 3–4). In keeping with other scholars who have studied hospital practices in nineteenth-century Canada, Shortt (1981) reports that historical records of lay midwives are often incomplete or unavailable. Historical writing on Canadian midwives has thus been limited, although there is a renewed interest in excavating documentary materials related to lay midwives and trained midwives and nurses who succeeded them (see Benoit 1991).

The nature of birth attendance in early Canada varied considerably. As the report of the task force on the implementation of midwifery in Ontario indicates, midwifery was established in Nova Scotia and Quebec. Midwives were an integral part of Mennonite communities in Manitoba, and in first-generation Japanese-Canadian communities in the lower mainland of British Columbia. Nevertheless, throughout Ontario and the western region, "women whose primary function was midwifery were rare." Instead, a "neighbour network" developed in North America, with neighbours assisting one another in child-birth (Mason 1987, 201–3; Edwards and Waldorf 1984). Lay midwives in pre-Confederation Canada were often affiliated with specific immi-grant groups (Canadian Broadcasting Corporation 1981). Cameron (1982, 243–9) provides a fictional account of native Indians attending a white woman in labour. Historical accounts indicate that native midwives assisted settlers and one another in the colony of British Columbia: "In the earliest days there were no trained nurses such as we know in 1945, and there were no hospitals. It was not considered necessary for a mother to go to a hospital for the birth of a child, and, further, it was not considered a matter for hospital attention. Children, in those days, were born in their homes – not in hospitals ... In Moodyville, a neighbour acted, assisted by an Indian woman, and at the Hastings Sawmill, and in Granville it was much the same ... Indian women never had mid-wives other than another Indian woman" (Matthews 1945).

A history of Pemberton, British Columbia, reports that native mid-wives assisted settlers in childbirth: "Babies were delivered by Indian mid-wives trained in their own traditional herb medicines, or by neighbours such as Mrs. Neill. The more prosperous or more nervous [women] preferred to travel to Vancouver several weeks ahead of time" (Decker et al. 1978, 241). The authors add that trained nurse-midwives were desired by women in the Pemberton area, and even-tually trained nurse-midwives affiliated with the Squamish Public Health Service practised there. By the beginning of the twentieth century, maternity cases in British Columbia were increasingly directed to two general hospitals and four or five maternity homes, although "dozens" of midwives attended women in labour at home (Matthews 1947). There are oral histories on frontier midwives and nurses in Western Canada, including Icelandic and other ethnically affiliated midwives. In some places women trained in nursing and midwifery worked with country doctors; sometimes neighbourhood women were the sole birth attendants (Rasmussen, Savage, and Wheeler 1976; Gahagan 1979, 1). Coburn (1974) concludes that community midwifery was essential, since few doctors practised in the colony.

Mason (1988) has studied traditional birth cultures in Canada. She notes that outside the more densely settled areas, women relied on one another for labour support. Women were discouraged from labouring alone. Female kin and neighbours often assisted in birth, providing what midwives today refer to as "continuity of care." A cardinal rule for midwives in this traditional birth culture "seems to have been to stay with the mother throughout the whole of her labour, to comfort her, and never to leave her by herself" (Mason 1988, 101). Parallels to modern community midwifery practice are evident: for example, women were encouraged to adopt various positions for delivery, and to move around during labour rather than being confined to the lithotomy position, or bedridden (Mason 1988, 102). She summarizes the traditional birth culture as offering several benefits: familiarity, companionship, various kinds of assistance to women and their families, provision for bedrest for women following birth, remedies, and birth attendance based more on reciprocity than on fee payments (see Mason 1987, 206). Strong-Boag (1988, 154), acknowledging that some concerns over unsafe midwifery practices might be justified, argues that these neighbourly midwives were valuable assets for many women: "Whatever their lack of professional qualifications, such women were cheap, potentially extremely helpful with domestic duties, and often reassuringly familiar when compared with their more scientific rivals ... as long as the pregnancy was normal and hospitals remained centres of infection and intervention, domestic surroundings and experienced, if unlicensed, care might be a very sensible solution."

The traditional birth culture stood for more than community customs in less settled areas. Mason (1988) found that where this culture was established, lower rates of maternal mortality were documented in midwife-attended home births than in physician-managed births. But even in the face of evidence favourable to some aspects of traditional birthing arrangements, "the proponents of more extensive medical involvement in birth had no interest in documenting the positive attributes of the traditional birth culture" (Mason 1988, 106). Possibilities for preserving the community-based culture gave way to an ethos of physician control of deliveries. Mason (1988, 111–12) uses the example of the Dionne quintuplets to highlight how physicians had positioned themselves as the most important caregivers. Although three of the Dionne quintuplets, born in 1934 in northern Ontario, were delivered by midwives, Dr. Dafoe delivered two of the babies and was given sole credit for his work. This credit was bolstered by his nomination for the Nobel Prize in medicine and his involvement in raising the quintuplets in an institution (see also Berton 1977).

The public health movement, showcasing medical attendance in tandem with nurses' involvement in maternity and infant care, began to accelerate after the First World War. Mason indicates that public health nurses helped to "propagandize" this system of birthing, a system that undermined women's confidence in birthing (Mason 1988, 212–15). This cultural emphasis on doctor-nurse management of birth was accompanied by technological experimentation, as well as a greater reliance upon caesarean section, the use of chloroform, and routine episiotomies. This experimentation did not lead to radical improvements in maternal mortality rates, and published findings suggested that many maternal and infant deaths were preventable (Mason 1988, 218–20). In North America, calls to reintroduce midwifery as part of an optimal health system fell from fashion and carried little weight in the early part of the twentieth century.

Midwifery care was not replaced so quickly in some areas of Canada. Midwives continued to practise in some outposts and in outport areas of Newfoundland. Benoit (1983, 1991) collected oral histories of empirical midwives in twentieth-century outports in Newfoundland. She explores the tradition of community self-help and folkways, along with the transformation of midwifery into obstetrical nursing. The Newfoundland midwives were typically forty years of age or older. Local midwives were generally well respected. Their practice was diversified, and ranged from birth attendance to bone-setting and veterinary care. In contrast to the fee-for-service practices of the professions, payment to community midwives was often made through bartering. The world of the outport midwife in Newfoundland was not entirely self-contained. Health threats to mothers and infants remained, and it was not uncommon for local midwives to accompany women to hospitals or nursing stations staffed by doctors or nurses. Some midwives also took formal training in Boston or other urban centres. Wendy Mitchinson points out that the movement toward hospital births in Canada was a feature of the twentieth century: "As late as 1939 more births occurred at home than in hospitals in the province of Ontario. For most of the nineteenth century few women would give birth in a hospital unless they absolutely had to. Hospitals were not particularly attractive places, and many refused to accept midwifery cases except in cases of emergency" (Mitchinson 1991, 183).

Coburn (1974) suggests that patriarchial ideology aided in the relegation of women to the domestic sphere, while professional ideology attracted trained nurses as allies with physicians against folk-healing and birth attendants. Historical accounts confirm the displacement of lay midwives by pioneer doctors and nurses. Increasingly, doctors were involved in home and hospital deliveries, occasionally assisting by telephone when travel proved impossible (see Burris 1967, 223–4). The exclusion of female birth attendants in the eighteenth and nineteenth centuries was accompanied by the refusal of medical schools in the United States and Canada to admit women (Donegan 1978, Strong-Boag 1979) to admit women. A female student who graduated from Queen's Medical School in Kingston, Ontario, faced hostility from male classmates (Smith 1980). Likewise, a woman applying for admission to the Royal College of Surgeons in Edinburgh in 1869 was ridiculed by her fellow students. There are more recent examples of dismissiveness and hostility directed toward female students in physics, psychology, and other disciplines (Ashley 1980, 16–17; Tuna 1989).

The exclusion of women from medical education can be linked with broader restrictions on women in nineteenth-century Canada. There was concern among some physicians that anatomy and physiology should not be taught to girls for fear of triggering hypochondria. The belief that women were by their nature ill-suited for competition and higher education was also reflected in this patriarchial differentiation of women and men (Mitchinson 1979, 16–17; 1991).

The professionalization of childbirth attendance in Canada has thus been placed in a critical framework of patriarchy and gender. Coburn sees the general ideology of women's inferiority as promoting work structures in which women's labour was auxiliary to men's work, voluntary (charitable), or poorly paid, and in which the material concerns of doctors and legislators were joined. The displacement of the lay midwife in Canada was not connected with the intrinsically superior power of medical and nursing attendants. Coburn (1974) adds that the intertwining of professionalism, sexism, and exclusion of women healers from lay practice and the barring of women from medical schools facilitated capital accumulation and industrialism.

The movement from the home to the hospital promoted structural disciplinary environments more conducive to industrialism.

Suzann Buckley maintains that the liaison between nurses and doctors in Canada, far from reflecting public preferences for professional attendance, stemmed from the professionals' interest in securing a monopoly over health-related services and from middle-class preferences for higher-ranking attendants. The securing of childbirth attendance also served to establish family medical practices for general practitioners. David Cayley (Canadian Broadcasting Corporation 1981) found that doctors obstructed attempts to establish midwifery certification and practice in Canada, and launched a "campaign of vilification" characterizing lay midwives as ignorant, dirty, and dangerous. As outlined earlier in this chapter, such campaigns were standard fare among European opponents of independent midwifery practice and training, and gained currency in North America as births became more medicalized. The strength of the opposition to midwifery stemmed in part from state prohibitions on improper practice, prohibitions that became entrenched in various statutes across Canada.

Law and the Containment of Midwifery

The ideology of professional attendance at birth and a growing number of surgical interventions were powerful forces in the movement to medically supervised hospital-based births. Legal prohibitions on midwifery practice also offered a deterrent to midwives practising without the protection of law. As Ward indicates, the movement of the state in regulating birth has varied considerably. In New France in the 1720s and 1730s, the Crown subsidized midwives trained in France. By 1788 the British required midwives practising in Montreal and Quebec City (and adjacent areas) to have a certificate. In 1879 the Quebec College of Physicians and Surgeons extended its control: in fact, approximately 95 per cent of midwifery licences were issued to male physicians and surgeons. In 1872, midwives in the City of Halifax were certified through a medical board while country midwives remained unregulated. In 1881, licensed physicians were legally empowered to practise midwifery. Peter Ward (1984, 7) reported that "even educated, well-qualified licensed midwives found themselves largely superseded, while those without training were confined to the countryside."

Biggs (1983, 22) saw legislation governing midwives in Upper Canada and eighteenth-century Ontario as a device enabling the exclusion of lay midwives: the 1795 Medical Act prohibited the practice of physic and surgery. This prohibition was reversed, however, by new legislation enacted in 1806; that legislation expressly protected midwifery practice: "nothing in this Act contained shall extend or be construed to extend to prevent any female from practising midwifery in any part of the Province, or to require such female to take out such license as aforesaid" (see Biggs 1983, 22).

Three bills to regulate or exclude domestic midwifery practice were defeated between 1845 and 1851. Nevertheless, medical influence was extended through the establishment of licensing powers, a system of registration, and medical education. With the increasing objections to midwifery – for undercutting doctors' fees, and for allegedly dangerous practices – midwifery attendance declined as doctors established practices in urban areas and as new legislation removed the protective status of female birth attendants set out in the 1806 legislation (Biggs 1983).

There was thus substantial opposition to suggestions that lay midwives could be trained and used in (remote) district nursing in nineteenth-century Canada. Attempts to import trained midwives were also resisted by some nineteenth- and twentieth-century Canadian physicians. Charlotte Hanington, the chief superintendent of the VON, hoped to assist prairie women by hiring approximately one hundred nurses from Britain. Buckley (1979, 145) notes that "the Canadian nurses were unreceptive ... sisterhood was narrowly defined in terms of the economic bonding of Canadian nurses. With the anticipated return of approximately 1,800 nurses from war work ... [the Canadian nurses] did not want to risk possible competition from group immigration of British nurses." Hanington's proposal and the objections to it followed much earlier attempts to restrict the practice of medicine in Upper Canada in 1795 to graduates of universities in the British Empire (Coburn 1974, 133–4).

In the United States there is no nationwide legislation to provide for midwifery services. Legislation regulating midwifery varies considerably: ten states prohibit the practice of lay midwifery, and in twenty-one states the status of lay midwives is unclear. In states that allow lay midwives to practise legally, a host of regulations can limit their practices: "attributes of state regulation which define the boundaries of practice, prohibit use of drugs, and require collaboration and backup by physicians are potentially inhibitory or hostile to lay midwifery. Having to depend on physicians to define which clients are low risk and experiencing normal pregnancies can be used as a device to restrict clientele, and having to rely on physician willingness to cooperate, consult, and provide support when complications arise or emergencies occur limits autonomy and can stifle the practice of lay midwives" (Butter and Kay 1988, 1168).

Opposition to lay midwives was generally tempered by the geographical distribution of the Canadian population. Until the early part of the twentieth century the population was primarily rural. The substantial distances that often separated inhabitants, compounded by inclement weather and rudimentary transportation, meant that birth attendance was often left to neighbouring women. Even where a clear preference for physican-attended births was stated, such limitations were recognized: one commissioner reporting to the Saskatchewan Services Survey Commission allowed that "while it is desirable to have women delivered by physicans, if possible in a maternity home, there are still numerous sections of the province that have no physician at all, and that, during the winter, are completely cut off from hospitals. In such regions, a nurse-midwife, that is a nurse trained in midwifery, could render invaluable services, *without encroaching upon the field of the physician*. A course would have to be devised for which the system practised in Alberta, England and other countries, would have to be consulted" (Sigerist 1944, emphasis added). Opposition to midwives was not characteristic of all doctors in pioneer Canada: there is evidence that relations between some doctors and midwives were amicable (Ward 1984, 13).

A controversial point is whether the monopoly status of Canadian doctors and nurses contributed to direct improvements in maternal and infant well-being. Buckley (1979, 132) established that maternal and infant mortality increased during this period of urbanization and replacement of the midwife. Shortt (1983–84) acknowledged that hospitals were often regarded as "gateways to death," and, where possible, were avoided by those who could afford home attendance and the general practice of physicians. It is farfetched to attribute declines in the rates of infant and maternal mortality to medicine per se when larger factors influence these rates. Besides improvements in sanitation, diet, and so forth, child-rearing customs affected the neonatal mortality rate.

The lack of resources for expectant mothers has been amply documented. Strong-Boag (1979, 154) notes that maternal deaths did not decrease between 1921 and 1938 in Canada, and concerns over preventable deaths led to many campaigns for better public health. Even these documented disparities in health between Canada and other countries did not lead to acceptance of midwifery among the medical profession: the "great majority" of doctors were unwilling to share birth attendance with midwives, and licensing was not made available to many practising midwives.

The transition from home births to hospital births involved an interstitial period in which domiciliary midwifery was practised extensively by public health nurses. In 1925, Coburn notes, 38,634 births occurred in VON hospitals or Red Cross outpost hospitals, whereas the VON attended 14,700 obstetrical cases at home (Coburn 1974, 150). Thus, approximately 27 per cent of births managed by the VON at this time were home births.

Domiciliary midwifery in Vancouver was praised for its safety. Nationwide, approximately 24,000 maternity cases were assisted by members of the VON, of which 5,000 were home births. Apparently, however, only a small minority at this time were managed by the nurse without the doctor present (Whitton 1945, 5, 27). Notwithstanding the work of public health nurses in attending home deliveries, the shift to hospital delivery was dramatic. It has been estimated that only 40 per cent of Canadian mothers delivered in hospital in 1939, and that 93 per cent delivered in hospital by 1959 (Cosbie 1969). The reasons underlying this shift from home to hospital deliveries include greater accessibility to hospitals and professional attendance, improved availability of services through provincial and federal funding of hospital construction, the development of medicare plans, and a cultural shift that promoted the skills of physicians and surgeons over those of midwives.

Midwifery in the United States

The hegemonic status of doctors in the management of childbirth also characterized developments in the United States (Starr 1982). The shift from lay practitioners, many of whom were women, in colonial America was gradual. Midwifery in eighteenth-century America was not subject to substantial formal regulation. Midwives were not regulated until the middle of the sixteenth century, when episcopal licensure ensured, among other things, that babies were baptized at birth (Donegan 1978). After 1776, many legislatures extended licensing powers to medical societies. These licensing powers usually exempted apothecaries, botanists, and midwives. In the Jacksonian period, however, women were no longer so dominant in healing.

Doctors mobilized against lay midwives. An ideology of protection of women from "unfeminine" work gained currency, and urban middle-class women began to choose physician attendance in childbirth between the mid-1700s and the Civil War (Starr 1982, 49; Donegan 1978, 4–5). In the nineteenth century, the campaign against "granny midwives" continued in the southern United States. In W. Eugene Smith's photographs of Maude Callen, a black nurse-midwife, the accompanying essay clearly favours nurse-midwives over traditional birth attendants. The nurse-midwife maintained aseptic conditions and had proper supplies – a blood-pressure gauge, cord ties, a stethoscope, and sterilized gloves. The distrust of lay midwives is unmistakable: "The new midwife had succeeded where the fast-disappearing 'granny' midwife of the South, armed with superstition and a pair of rusty scissors, might have killed both mother and child" (Smith 1951, 135). Implicit in the pictorial essay is a sense that with their training, versatility, and commitment these nurse-midwives met many unmet needs, not least of all among the poor.

In the early nineteenth century, fatalities attributed to unlicensed midwives attracted newspaper coverage. Concerns over high rates of childbirth-related deaths culminated in 1933 in a major report on maternal mortality in New York City. The recommendation that proper training of midwives should be encouraged was largely disregarded (New York Academy of Medicine 1933). The lay midwife was seen as competing with physicians. Nurse-midwives were valued by obstetricians for their assistance in childbirth (Starr 1982, 223). Even if midwives could circumvent licensing restrictions, they could not collect from Blue Shield plans, and their patients could not collect under indemnity insurance plans (Starr 1982, 333). Like their European counterparts, American physicians were successful in establishing clinical instruction programs in which medical students viewed the birth of babies. This was not a wholesale movement away from midwifery. Litoff (1978, 20) points to the proliferation of dispensaries and hospitals in which demonstrative midwifery was acceptable. Demonstrative midwifery required that the birth attendant abandon the norm of modesty and view the woman's genitals during labour, birth, and the post-partum period. Manual examinations of women by male physicians were permitted in the mid-nineteenth century but visual examination of a woman's genitals was forbidden (Ward 1984, 14). The innovation of "demonstrative midwifery" by Dr. James White in Buffalo in 1850 was widely debated but eventually became established (Litoff 1978, 20; Drachman 1979).

As in England and Canada, medical opinion in the United States was divided over midwifery. Some American physicians spoke for midwives in the late nineteenth and early twentieth centuries. For example, in 1884 Dr. T.H. Manley argued for the utilization of trained midwives. Seeing midwifery and medicine as complementary, Manley suggested that midwives could utilize physicians in difficult cases, while physicians could respect the skill of "the properly qualified midwife" (Litoff 1978, 21–2). Concerns were expressed over the supposed dangerousness of midwives, the folly of investing money in training midwives (when medicine and nursing could be fostered), and the need to incorporate midwifery practice by law as a branch of medicine practised exclusively by the medical profession (Litoff 1978, 22). The controversy over midwifery led to proposals for nurse-midwifery, a term coined in 1914 by Dr. Fred Taussig, a Missouri physician. Taussig believed that midwifery training should be restricted to nursing graduates. The nurse-midwife would receive specialized training in obstetrics, and in Taussig's view would be the best possible complement to medical attendance at births (see Litoff 1978, 22–3).

The midwifery debate in the United States brings forward many themes discussed earlier in this chapter. First, there were few avenues leading to training and certification for midwives, even in late nineteenth-century America. Some programs that did exist were clearly substandard, although a number of midwifery colleges and schools were established. Litoff (1978, 136) concludes that at the turn of the twentieth century, programs for midwives "were highly inadequate." A second feature of the American debate was the debate within the medical profession and public health agencies. The anti-midwife campaign reached its zenith between 1910 and 1920. Some physicians believed that midwifery interfered with the proper development of obstetrics and posed a hazard to the public. Conversely, some public health officials believed that midwives, properly trained and supported, could lower maternal and infant mortality rates. These proponents of midwifery drew on European data in support of midwifery as well as American studies of midwifery programs (Litoff 1978, 136–9).

The hegemonic status of physicians in birth in many parts of America was not a boon for all Americans. Sullivan and Weitz indicate that recorded rates of mortality and morbidity increased as physicians displaced midwives and instrumental deliveries became commonplace. They add that with formal development of medicine, certain groupings were disadvantaged. Medical training was accompanied by higher standards of admission, longer programs, and greater tuition costs, and few schools were accessible to "blacks, women, or working-class students." Consequently, birth attendance shifted away from midwives and toward control by wealthier white males (Sullivan and Weitz 1988, 17). The fusion of medicine and birth continued, despite published accounts of unwanted and potentially dangerous interventions during birth. These interventions – artificially delaying birth so as to allow physicians to attend; strapping women to delivery tables (sometimes without medical or nursing attendance); routine shaving of the pubic area; and injuries attributed to forceps deliveries – were often countered by those enthralled with the importance of keeping the "obstetrical field" sterile and protected, and by the belief that these complaints were "in the mothers' heads" (Sullivan and Weitz 1988, 24–5).

Nowhere has the midwife been displaced without controversy. That controversy is very much alive today in many parts of the world (see Kitzinger 1988). The great campaigns to dislodge midwives – in the United States, between 1850 and 1930 and in the early to mid-twentieth century in Canada, for example – have attracted opponents as well as advocates of midwifery. It appears that today a renewed appreciation of the politics underlying midwifery is gaining strength. Arguments that medical supervision and routine technological intervention are in the public interest seem facile and lacking in empirical proof. That said, midwifery is not gaining strength worldwide; some commentators suggest that midwives as a group are declining in influence in Europe, for instance. The following section provides a selective look at midwifery and birthing practices in different cultures.

CROSSCULTURAL PERSPECTIVES ON MIDWIFERY

Midwifery is not only a local practice in many countries, but has lodged as a worldwide organization or set of organizations. The International Confederation of Midwives (ICM) is based in London, England. The ICM represents sixty-one countries worldwide, including Canada. The ICM holds a triennial congress. The 1993 Congress was held in Vancouver, Canada. The ICM and many other world bodies, including the United Nations and the World Health Organization, have been largely favourable to midwifery practice. As set out below, there are many differences in the ways midwifery is practised across cultures, and there is a growing sense of urgency with respect to persistent patterns of preventable maternal and infant deaths and injuries, especially in the developing world. As we will see, there is also concern that the principles of continuity of care for expectant mothers and a varied sphere of practice for qualified midwives might be compromised.

Cross-cultural variations in midwifery practice and birth practices in general have long been recorded. Midwives are variously called *sage-femme* (France and Quebec), *dukun bagi* (Java), *nana* (Jamaica), and *partera* (Hispanic countries). Other names include *comadrona, bidan,* and *dai* (Cosminsky 1976). Traditional midwives are almost always women, although there are cultures in which male midwives have practised. Laderman (1983) describes a male *bidan* in a Malaysian hamlet as "a great rarity." His practice ceased when a female village midwife moved to his hamlet. Hart (1965, 22–3) reported that males began practising midwifery in the rural Philippines after 1963. Male midwives were referred to as *sibulan*.

Several themes become evident when one examines cross-cultural materials on midwifery and childbirth. First, anthropological studies have captured the diversity of childbirth practices in various cultures. In many non-industrialized cultures a variety of beliefs and customs have been recorded. These include dietary restrictions and proscriptions concerning those who may attend births. In some cultures, husbands are expected to be absent during the birth; in others the absence of the father is seen as a portent of misfortune for the newborn child. Birthing positions likewise vary from the standard lithotomy position (on one's back) in western medical practice to a variety of birthing positions, including squatting, on all fours, on birthing stools, and using ropes or poles for support. The complexity of this subject is evident not only between cultures but also within some cultures. Research on the Rogai of South Vietnam, for instance, showed that women deliver their babies using a variety of gravitational aids: birthing stools, ropes, vines, and poles for support (Lee 1972, 40).

One issue in the modern debate over obstetrics and midwifery is the use of technology for control purposes. Critics of the unnecessary use of obstetrical technology claim that a variety of surgical measures such as episiotomy and caesarean section do more serve than medical purposes; they also help to consolidate and reinforce medical power during childbirth. There have been shifts in this debate, however. Women's associations lobbied for the use of scopolamine (a narcotic and analgesic, also known as "twilight sleep") in 1914 and 1915, whereas some modern feminists lobby for the option of unmedicated births:

The twilight sleep movement helped change the definition of birthing from a natural home event, as it was in the nineteenth century, to an illness requiring hospitalization and physician attendance. Parturient feminists today, seeking fully to experience childbirth, paradoxically must fight a tradition of drugged, hospital-controlled births, itself the partial result of a struggle to increase women's control over their bodies (Leavitt 1980, 164).

A number of writers have linked the growth of technological approaches to childbirth with the alienation of mothers. Recourse to routine induction of labour (in the absence of a sound medical reason) has been associated to some extent with professional convenience (Cartwright 1979). For some, the act of accepting pain relief in labour alters the essential quality of birth, reducing the woman receiving medication to "a passive thing" (McMillan 1982, 133).

Variations in Infant Mortality Rates

The cycle of birth and death has changed dramatically in modern times. In developed countries, the average lifespan has lengthened dramatically compared with earlier times: "'It is not uncommon, I have frequently been told,' Adam Smith soberly noted, 'in the Highlands of Scotland for a mother who has borne twenty children not to have two alive.' The poor died freely, in unrecorded numbers, but even men of means thought long life a stroke of unexpected luck" (cited in Gay 1970, 21). High rates of infant mortality were a feature of early life in colonial Canada, and maternal mortality was also a threat (Backhouse 1991). Mitchinson (1991, 224–5) notes that puerperal fever – "infection originating in the birth canal, which can spread throughout the body, causing septicaemia and eventual death" – was especially common in the nineteenth century.

If the ideal of a "best birth" and long life have become cultural expectations in western countries, the same cannot be said of many other countries. It is estimated that every year half a million women die of childbirth-related problems (including complications from abortion, infection, and other aspects of birth). In many countries, women are likely to suffer from too many closely spaced pregnancies, compounded by giving birth at too early an age. These dangers are often exacerbated by inadequate sanitation and hygiene, and a weak health-care infrastructure. In the World Health Organization's film *Why Did Mrs. X Die?*, the viewer is shown several points at which a mother's life could have been saved if adequate resources had been made available to her. A report issued in 1986 confirmed the extent to which women's and infants' health is compromised in many countries: "Some progress has already been made in reducing infant mortality, but the differential in maternal mortality between rich and poor countries is among the highest observed in public health, reports WHO (World Health Organization). Eighty-five per cent of the world's births take place in developing countries but these same countries suffer 95 per cent of the world's *infant deaths,* and a terrible 99 per cent of all *maternal deaths.* WHO figures also show that more women die in India in 1 month than die in all of North America, Europe and Australia in 1 year" (Anonymous 1986, 53; emphasis in original).

Beyond the problem of direct assistance in childbirth, international attention is increasingly focused on the status of women, especially in the developing world. Illiteracy and discrimination contribute to health problems among women (Royston and Armstrong 1989, 45–74). There are efforts within many developing countries to secure better services and legal rights for women. For example, midwives associated with the Movement for Humanitarian Birth (*Movimiento Pro-Parto Humanizado*) have outlined ten "fundamental rights for the pregnant woman." These rights include free prenatal care and education, active participation in all stages of birth, attention and assistance by professionals, and the right to choose where to give birth and those who may attend the birth. Concern over the half-million women who die or are injured as a result of pregnancy or childbirth-related problems has led the International Confederation of Midwives and others to favour a stronger role for the midwife. This role would include community education, administration of various health-related projects and resources, and greater access to research and education (International Confederation of Midwives 1987, 18–22).

There is substantial controversy over the part played by medical science in reducing infant and maternal mortality, and the influence of improved hygiene, sanitation, and diet (McKinlay and McKinlay 1976). Regardless, in Europe and other industrialized countries there has been a great reduction since the eighteenth century in the proportion of children who die in childbirth or in the first few years of childhood. Historical records from parishes in Finland, for example, indicate that the infant mortality rate in 1809 in one rural parish was 970 per 1,000 births (during a typhoid epidemic). In 1881, the rate was 375 per 1,000 births. Many infants who died between one and six months of age suffered from gastric illnesses or contagious diseases, and breast-feeding provided greater protection against these illnesses (see Lithell 1981). Higher rates of infant mortality within western societies have been noted for black infants in the United States (Yankauer 1979; Seager and Olson 1986, section 10) and for native infants in Canada. A greater incidence of low birth weight and infant mortality in the Northwest Territories in 1972 was noted by Smith (1976). Mortality rates among reserve Indians in Ontario in 1898 were three times the provincial rate (Weaver 1972, 43).

There is a substantial difference in birth rates in comparison with Third World countries. Studies early in this century recorded what are today regarded as high rates of infant mortality. Two studies noted by Kitzinger (1978, 75, 107) address miscarriages in a South African tribe between 1929 and 1935. One study found that 12.5 per cent of pregnancies in another African village resulted in miscarriage, while 28 per cent of newborns did not survive to maturity. Even in modern times comparatively high rates of infant mortality have been documented in non-industrialized areas. The authors of a 1973

UNICEF report estimated that 17.6 per cent of babies born in an Arabian community died in their first year. By age two, this statistic exceeded 23 per cent (Eickelman 1984, 126, 181).

Dangers to the mother during labour, delivery, and post-partum were also evident. In the Yucatan, birth attendants are vigilant in watching for placental retention, which can cause maternal deaths (Jordan 1981). In many cultures maternal deaths are attributed to supernatural powers, including witchcraft. Smith-Bowen (1964, ch. 14) wrote a poignant account of the death of her friend Amara, a woman from a bush tribe in Africa. Her friend's death revealed the clash between reliance on western medicine as a life-saving measure and the tribe's cultural belief in powers of magic. Others have noted the belief in spirits as causes of death in childbirth. In Malaysia, the *badi mayat* – an evil spirit or principle believed to exist in a human corpse – was associated with the wasting away of an infant (Laderman 1982, 95–102). The author attributed the infant death to a misdiagnosis at a medical clinic.

One former nurse I spoke with in the early 1980s had assisted Bedouin women in Saudi Arabia in the late 1950s and early 1960s. She recounted one instance in which western medicine was well received by the tribe.

I suppose it was about eight o'clock in the morning and I went out to this infant that had been born between four and five a.m. The doctor had delivered it. It was a Friday, a religious holiday, and since it was a day of rest he had gone off to Kwaittown; as far as he was concerned it was a fairly standard delivery. It was the first time I've taken a pulse that I couldn't count quickly enough: the pulse rate was so high. The infant's temperature went off the thermometer, over 108 degrees. I had never seen anything like this, and what I did in panic (not through skill), was to move the mother and the family into the jeep and we drove across the desert to a medical clinic which happened to be air-conditioned. I sponged the infant down and his temperature came down nicely. I was scared to take him out again ... I waited until the sun went down to take him to a doctor at a neighbouring oil company. This was the seventh baby this women had birthed, and every one had died on the first day of birth. Their metabolic rate followed the sun's temperature ... and of course they would die once the sun was out ... We kept this seventh child in the air-conditioned room and gradually exposed it to the outside. Eventually this infant's system just corrected itself and it grew, it coped. This made an incredible impact on the local people.

A common theme in reconstructing childbirth ritual in Third World countries is the control women usually exert in birth attendance. This control extended to reproduction generally, including contraception and abortion. Some scholars conclude that men were excluded from these matters or involved only marginally (Oakley 1976, 19–23). In some Philippine villages fathers were expected to be present, while in some northern India locales fathers were excluded from childbirth (Whiting and Whiting 1979, 112). Indian fathers in Guatemala were expected to assist their wives in childbirth by bracing them in a supported squatting delivery position (Maynard 1974, 90).

This theme has been qualified by other accounts pointing to the folk perception of women as dangerous in a number of cultures (Chodorow 1971, 274). Childbirth ritual has been specifically interpreted as devaluing women while consolidating a medical model of technologically based, professionally managed birth.

Traditional Practices and the Medicalization of Birth

The medicalization of childbirth is evident in Third World countries and elsewhere. Increasingly, traditional midwives, many of whom apprenticed with other lay midwives and practised in their villages for decades, are being displaced in favour of nurses trained in obstetrical nursing or midwifery, or by physicians. The traditional reliance on touch, on amulets, and so forth has likewise been overshadowed by technological machinery and the role of technicians in medicalized antenatal, postnatal, and labour and delivery stages. Record-keeping is emphasized, registration of births and deaths is required by law, and control over licensure and training is formally vested in such government bodies as departments of health.

Traditional midwives in Malaysia – *bidan kampung* – have been trained in principles of hygiene, sterile techniques, and family-planning. Home deliveries have tended to shift to formally trained nurse-midwives. There has been some degree of adaptation on the part of government-trained midwives to local customs. Nevertheless, the legislation requiring midwives to be registered (and the lack of registration procedures for new village midwives) means that village midwifery is likely to disappear when the current *bidans* retire. The *bidan kampung* are responsible for instruction in breast-feeding (or the proper preparation of formula) and family planning, but not for assistance in labour and delivery (Chen 1977).

Western influences on traditional birth practices are not entirely irresistible. Opposition to western medical practices has been noted among rural women in Guatemala, Malaysia, Papua New Guinea, and the Yucatan (Cosminsky 1976; Chen 1978; Jordan 1980). Nevertheless, there has been a clear movement away from home delivery and toward hospital or clinic deliveries in many Third World countries. The shift toward medical management of births has benefited some infants and mothers through the availability of modern equipment and improved training of birth attendants in nutrition, sepsis, and careful management of labour, delivery, and post-partum complications.

McClain's (1975) fieldwork in Ajijic – forty kilometres from Guadalajara, Mexico – revealed a variegated system of maternity care. Women delivered at home with traditional birth attendants (*parteras*) or with an attending physician. Increasingly, women in Ajijic delivered in hospitals. Accompanying this trend away from home deliveries was a decline in the number of practising *parteras*, coupled with the aging of two of the three practising midwives.

There are numerous instances of resistance to the western model and the incorporation of valuable aspects of western medicine (asepsis, more nourishing diets, encouragement of earlier breastfeeding to provide colostrum to newborns) with traditional rituals (McClain 1975). A detailed biography of Jesuita Aragon, a senior midwife in Los Vegas, a small community in northern New Mexico, captures the incorporation of traditional healing practices with modern principles of hygiene and professional attendance. At the time of writing, folk beliefs in supernatural elements coexisted to some degree with the use of sterilized equipment, procedures for emergency transfers to hospital, and instruction by nurses (Buss 1980). Traditional Hispanic midwives have nevertheless fallen in numbers, and it seems more appropriate to speak of the replacement or displacement of folk healers and midwives by professional healers (see Brack 1976). One point of commonality between latter-day and modern lay midwifery is a spritual dimension in maternity care. Black "granny midwives" in the southern United States sang spirituals during meetings with nurses. The advent of formal midwifery instruction was not always opposed by the granny midwives, and in some instances it was welcomed (Campbell 1946, 23–4). Source materials on the retention of African practices by Southern black midwives include documentation of practices in folk midwifery. The authors claim that many of these folk practices have been adopted by modern obstetricians to improve birth outcomes for mothers and infants (Conklin et al., 1983, 79). Hull (1979, 316) found that midwives in rural Java believed that colostrum was contaminated, used septic bamboo blades to sever the umbilical cord, and manually removed the placenta, sometimes causing serious infections. A Western-trained midwife observed four village midwives in India engaging in harmful practices such as performing vaginal examinations after touching cow dung (thus producing tetanus and other infections), rupturing membranes with fingernails, exerting manual pressure on the fundus (see also Dole 1974, 24 regarding Peruvian midwives), and a cultural prohibition on "cold" foods and substances that led to dehydration and ketosis poisoning (Tyson 1984, 5–6).

Some researchers have disagreed with favourable assessments of the work of traditional midwives in Third World countries. Midwives in rural Vietnam were described as lacking precise knowledge of the management of complicated deliveries. Their ineptitude could lead to "disaster" for mothers or their infants (Coughlin 1965, 213). Midwives in Mexico were perceived as not being knowledgeable about diagnosis of pregnancy, midwifery techniques in uncomplicated deliveries, and appropriate responses for complicated deliveries when a doctor was unavailable to them. Moreover, criticisms of indigenous midwives have emerged from their home countries – for example, in the Philippines (Velimirovic and Velimirovic 1981, 91–2)

Other beliefs in traditional cultures clash with medical science. McClain's (1975, 40–1) study of birth in a small Mexican community touched on the folk belief that a father's blood-drop created female embryos, while a mother's created male embryos. Congenital deformities, spontaneous abortions, and stillbirths were attributed to factors external to the mother, not to genetically determined abnormalities.

It has been generally reported that septic procedures by traditional midwives in tropical countries contributed to serious infections (da Cruz 1969, 354). One program in rural Bangladesh was designed to incorporate some traditional practices with principles of hygiene and adequate diet. The attendance of the traditional midwife, the *dai*, was supervised by paramedical staff and complemented by a local clinic consisting of a physician and other paramedics. The custom of withholding breast-feeding for three to five days after birth did not allow the newborn to receive colostrum (which aids the developing immune response system). Education regarding appropriate supplementary feeding when breast-feeding continues into the sixth month was also carried out, as was instruction in sanitation and hygiene to reduce the substantial numbers of children dying of post-partum tetanus and sepsis during infancy (see Bhatia 1981, 70–1).

High rates of infant mortality have thus been linked with inferior skills of traditional birth attendants. However, it has not been established that decreases in infant and maternal mortality rates are attributable primarily to advances in the medical and nursing sciences. A wider context of health care is needed. One researcher studying birth practices and infant mortality on a Guatemalan *finca* (plantation) commented: "The main causes of this problem do not lie in the birth practices themselves, but in the poor nutritional and health state of the mothers, the poverty and the larger socioeconomic problems of the *finca* population" (Cosminsky 1977, 101). Research in American cities has likewise documented a positive correlation between poverty (and race) and infant mortality. It is generally accepted that many deaths of neonates (babies under twenty-eight days old) are caused by congenital factors, whereas post-neonatal mortality is more likely to be associated with low income of mothers (Brooks 1980, 2–11).

The crosscultural evidence helps to identify cultural patterns that promote high-quality midwifery care, or to restrict it. Jeffery and her associates studied childbearing and other events in northern India. They found that health policy had to some extent followed a grass-roots strategy of using *dais*, traditional birth attendants, as part of maternity care. The authors pointed out that many other developing countries have not taken up recommendations for similar programs, and that even in northern India there are unsafe practices that endure in the care of mothers and infants, as well as official limitations in offering the best possible service. They conclude that, in practice, "the state is demonstrating no firm commitment to maternal medical services, either of the conventional clinical kind or the so-called grass-roots version put forward as an alternative. Commercial and other interests prevail, thereby reducing official policy to empty rhetoric" (Jeffrey, Jeffrey, and Lyon 1989, 220).

The diversity of birth ritual and belief systems in the countries mentioned above is not absent in more affluent western countries. There is no question that there has been an entrenchment of obstet-rics and technological monitoring and management of childbirth, such that what Arney (1983, 9) calls "obstetrical space" has been extended. Davis-Floyd (1990) is critical of the misrepresentation of American "obstetrical rituals" as progressive and desirable. Instead, these rituals help to establish a patriarchal system of birthing in which women's bodies are often treated mechanistically. Birth as a natural process is thus often displaced, recast as a perilous journey that must be monitored by obstetrical staff. Davis-Floyd's critique of the medical model of birth makes an important link between seem-ingly benign interventions and wider structures of control in Amer-ican society.

There are variations within cultures that are predominantly but not wholly dependent on professional maternity care. Hazell (1974) found that many of the women giving birth at home in California used a variety of birthing positions, including supported squatting and delivery on all fours. He noted that in many non-European countries the upright birthing position and the side-lying positions were commonly used, while the lithotomy position remains standard practice in western obstetrics. Odent provided data favouring the use of supported squatting delivery positions, and suggesting that episiotomy rates can be reduced through such initiatives. Of 898 births in Pithiviers in 1980, only 8 per cent required episiotomies; the rate of caesarean section was 5 per cent (Odent 1981, 7–15). Midwives have also studied alternatives to medical interventions – for example, methods for managing shoulder dystocia (Meenan et al. 1992).

The meeting of east and west is captured in the following excerpt from a letter sent by a British Columbia midwife working in the former Soviet Union to another British Columbia midwife. The writer, who was part of an exchange program involving American and Russian midwives, commented on outmoded rituals of routine enemas, perineal shaves, artificial rupture of membranes, and use of the lithotomy position in state-supported maternity hospitals (see also Shea 1991). She described a "deep revolution" in birthing protocols in a private hospital in St. Petersburg:

We decided to do a presentation [to staff]. We would try and show (and back up with statistics) alternative techniques. We showed slides of women birthing upright, or on their sides, or on all fours. And a long, long discussion ensued ... Soon after the discussion I went to the labour-delivery floor. A few of our midwives were there because a woman was in labour, and actually delivering the baby when I arrived ... at least 3 doctors were in the room – they had been at the presentation – plus 3 [Russian] midwives and 2 of "us" ... [The birth attendants] were given permission to leave the woman on the bed, not on the delivery table. She was allowed to deliver on her side, no drugs, no episiotomy. The baby was quietly placed on the mother's belly and she held her baby for at least 20 minutes before the baby exam had to happen ...

Soon afterwards, another woman hit second stage and the Russian midwife and doctor working with her got excited and said, "We're doing it that way!" So another woman delivered on the bed, in a semi-sitting position, the boy placed on her belly, etc. [The staff] were grinning from ear to ear. Whether or not anyone was conscious of it, I suspect the sense of empowerment hit everybody and some sort of deep revolution is happening at this hospital ... Later that afternoon, another woman delivered her baby in a quasi-squat on the bed. It was a complete, "hands-off" birth. It is obvious that the staff at this hospital have reached a point of no return ... (letter from Michelle Buchmann to Barb Ray, 3 December 1992)

Jordan's (1980) award-winning study of childbirth practices in four countries pointed to significant differences in childbirth management between western nations: specifically, the Dutch approach retained domiciliary deliveries and discouraged routine medication, whereas Swedish practitioners relied on painkillers and hospital-based obstetrics. Home birth is not only a feature of contemporary Third World countries. In Holland, for example, approximately one-third of births occur at home (Brook 1980, 7). Nevertheless, the list of contraindications to home birth in Holland has increased over time, while the percentage of births at home has slowly but steadily decreased in recent years (Kloosterman 1981, 9–24). A hallmark of Dutch birthing policy is the reliance on midwifery assistance in birth, whether at home or in hospitals or clinics.

Midwifery in Japan and China

The majority of published works on cross-cultural midwifery practices pertain to Europe, North America, and Third World countries. A sense of midwifery practice and of kinship practices surrounding birth in the Orient is provided by some recent studies. For example, Kitahara (1982) reported that midwives in Japan must be licensed and, as in Denmark, must practice in hospital settings. Bradley-Low (1984) viewed birth in Japan as hospital-oriented, technological, and medically dominated, with some counter-trends in domiciliary and clinic midwifery practice. In her detailed observations of health care customs in Japan, Jacobson (1974, 108) drew attention to the incorporation of scientific medicine with established kinship relations. Specifically, the practice of *satogaeri* – returning to the natal home for delivery of a first child – is fairly common, and stands in some contrast to the usual practice in Canada of women delivering in their own locality (Jacobson 1974, 108). The blend of modernity and tradition is also evident in the frequent use of the pregnancy sash (*iwata-obi*), which is thought to promote easier delivery by restricting the size of the fetus, and in the reliance on obstetricians, hospitals, and clinics (Ohnuki-Tierney 1984, 181–8).

The global movement toward professionalized attendance in childbirth is apparent in China and Japan. This movement appears most pronounced in urban centres. In the early 1970s, it was reported that Chinese babies born in cities were usually delivered in hospitals, with doctors supervising the births. Babies born in the countryside were delivered at home with the assistance of midwives. Anaesthesia was not routinely used for uncomplicated deliveries (Sidel 1973, 59–61).

CONCLUSION

Cross-cultural birthing practices reflect considerable variation in birthing customs and the role of the midwife. Crucial to an evaluation of midwifery development in Canada, however, is the finding that only 9 of 210 nations studied by the World Health Organization made no provision for midwifery service. Canada was one of these nine nations, and the only major industrialized nation without established midwifery services in the infrastructure of national birth attendance. The history of midwives in Europe reveals important variations: the promotion of scientific midwifery in France and Germany, for instance, contrasts with the general absence of publicly sponsored midwifery instruction and government regulation in England.

The conflict over midwifery in British North America reflected many of these European concerns. Much of the literature on midwifery in Canada is critical of the takeover of birth by physicians and the displacement of midwifery. Nevertheless, serious consideration must be given to benefits that have accrued from medical research, nursing, and medical training. These benefits include a stronger knowledge base on pregnancy, birth, and child development, and the translation of this knowledge into improved clinical care.

The point remains, however, that these benefits are not clearly predicated on medical dominance in childbirth. Substantial research has been undertaken and clinical programs have been established in many countries worldwide in conjunction with developed midwifery programs. Further work in understanding Canada's anomalous policy on midwifery could be connected with Lipset's interpretation of greater deference to élites in Canada and the identification of deference as a trait in Canadian political culture (Lipset 1986, 138). Despite the renaissance of community midwifery and demands for direct entry midwifery training (autonomous midwifery), less than 1 per cent of deliveries in North America are planned home births.

Not all jurisdictions in Canada and the United States expressly prohibit the practice of community midwifery or nurse-midwifery (Barrington 1985, 40–1; Sallomi, Pallow, and McMahon 1981). The regulation of midwives in North America also varies from province to province. The variations in provincial statutes lend support to the historically specific nature of states, as opposed to a monolithic view of state regulation of midwives. Federal, provincial, and state levels are not uniform in their statutes and may vary in their enforcement of these statutes.

Historical accounts of midwifery in Canada have generally high-lighted the struggle between men and women evidenced by the exclusion of women from the universities, and the ideology of a "proper sphere" of reproduction and domesticity (Cook and Mitchinson 1976). The fault-finding remarks by some physicians about midwifery practice are misplaced, especially those concerning the competency of trained midwives practising as members of an autonomous or semi-autonomous profession. As this chapter has indicated, the general rejection of independent midwifery practice in North America stands in contrast to its acceptance in many other countries. The review of midwifery practice in Canada in the next chapter provides additional support for the viability of regulated midwifery practice in home and hospital settings. It also strikes a strong note of caution in connection with opting for regulation at any cost if historical patterns of denigrating midwives are to be avoided.

CHAPTER FOUR

"To Be with Woman": Midwifery Practice in Canada

The autonomous midwife – frequently self-trained – is a major anomaly in Canadian health care ... Over 200 midwives ... have provided care for thousands of women in their homes over the past 15 years in Canada. This is a situation that organized medicine, nursing and properly trained midwives should not contemplate with satisfaction.

Robert A.H. Kinch, "Midwifery and Home Births"

Women in our post-industrial culture are effectively captive in childbirth. The zoo may be run on scientific principles, the keepers may be considerate and may pride themselves on the good condition of the animals and the low mortality rate. Visiting times may be frequent and the zoo may be a friendly, welcoming place. In the confines of the cage there may be space to move about, and those in charge may have tried to replicate the natural habitat. Yet captivity restrains and dictates the behavior of the captives.

Sheila Kitzinger, Homebirth

INTRODUCTION

In Canada there is a tremendous controversy over the implementation of midwifery. This chapter presents a detailed examination of midwifery practice and birth outcomes, using Canadian data in conjunction with studies from other countries. Before moving to this discussion of midwifery practice – in home births and in hospital settings – it is necessary to review how the research was conducted.

Community midwifery has endured since the early 1970s, but it has not flourished. The Midwives' Association of British Columbia (MABC) lobbies for legalized, autonomous midwifery and appropriate guidelines for midwifery practice. They consult with sympathetic medical and nursing practitioners, and only a few births out of thousands assisted by community midwives in Canada have resulted in criminal prosecution or prosecutions for violations of the British Columbia Medical Practitioners Act. Although there are comparatively few prosecutions, community midwifery is marginalized and illegal. Out-of-hospital births comprise less than 1 per cent of births in British Columbia (and nationwide). Community midwives are unable to bill for their services through the provincial medical services plan, and they do not have established hospital privileges. Community midwives are also more likely than medical personnel to be prosecuted for criminal negligence causing death. They are also subject to the quasi-criminal charge under the Medical Practitioners Act of practising medicine without a licence.

Community midwifery in Canada illustrates the structural limits placed on female birth attendants working outside the norm of professionally accredited, hospital-situated childbirth. For the past 20 years a debate over home birth – and more generally, midwifery – has been evident in Canada and other industrialized countries. This debate addresses several issues: maternal and infant wellbeing throughout pregnancy, delivery, and the postnatal stage; women's control over pregnancy and childbirth; and personal liberty and the overreaching powers of the state (including the institution of the hospital and the powers allotted to the professions). There is concern over the increased use of childbirth technology in labour and delivery, and what some regard as the alienation of health-care practitioners from their direct work with women (Arney 1982; Ruzek 1991; Kargar 1990).

Community midwifery emphasizes the decentralized nature of childbirth attendance, along with the more personal relationship between the community midwife and her constituency. Community midwifery has in general become better integrated with international associations, and more concerned with education, certification, and standards of practice. A case in point was the founding of the British Columbia School of Midwifery in Vancouver in 1985. Accredited in Washington state, the school offered a theoretically based curriculum along with opportunities for preceptorships (clinical experience in midwifery) in Holland, England, Jamaica, Germany, and the American state of Georgia). The tenuous legal status of midwives in British Columbia and the costs of operating a school without government support led to the suspension of school operations in 1987. This decision by the school board was seen as a temporary one, until such time as midwives achieved a more secure legal and clinical footing in the province.

COMMUNITY MIDWIFERY
IN CANADA

This section focuses on a study of attempted home births, primarily in British Columbia and Ontario. Where possible, reference is made to midwives' practices in other provinces and regions. The community midwife network in British Columbia is complex. Most midwives have learned their skills through a mixture of apprenticeship with senior midwives, their own experience, and reading, and some have moved into community midwifery after completing formal nursing requirements. The dichotomy between the traditional midwife and the professional midwife seems more appropriate for non-westernized societies, in which there may be substantial gaps in literacy, formal education, knowledge of hygiene, and birth management between the two groupings.

Empirical Training and the Midwifery School

One development in the community midwifery movement has been the extension of formal instruction into the movement. A full year of academic training was recently completed sub rosa by seventeen students through a midwifery school established in Vancouver by local community midwives and some of their supporters (Anderson 1986, 11). The academic phase, paid for by the students, staffed by midwives, and examined by midwives with international training, is followed by a clinical phase of preceptorship. While many of the new community midwives have not completed formal nursing requirements, a number of British Columbia midwives are either registered in (or are eligible to join) the Registered Nurses' Association of British Columbia. One practising community midwife expressed her ambivalence toward formal nursing training in childbirth: "The nursing was a mixed blessing. Nursing gave me a lot of the skills. I was comfortable giving injections, comfortable with catheterizations, with taking blood pressure and pulse, just those basic nursing skills that a midwife apprentice has to learn. And it can be difficult learning those skills. The thing that was really difficult for me was that even though I basically knew that women could birth babies, and birth them graciously and have them at home, it took me a long time to understand that on a gut level, and to really believe, yes, that women could give birth."

Against the norm of professionalized nursing, situated in the hospital and supervised by physicians, some nurses have opted for community midwifery practice. Midwives have nevertheless sought out other sources of training. Some out-of-province midwives report attending workshops as a form of instruction. A Manitoba community midwife noted: "After those first four births I went and took a very good workshop in Vancouver. I invested money and bought books and equipment and felt a little more like I knew what I was doing ..." (see Yusuf 1984). Another example is a Master of Midwifery (M.A.) program under development (in 1993) at Thames Valley University and Queen Charlotte's Hospital in London. Five Canadian midwives began this program in 1993. This said, the overall historical pattern of discouraging midwifery as a distinct, legally recognized profession continues in many provinces, except for Ontario and Alberta (Williams 1991).

Teamwork

A general principle is that community midwives prefer to assist in labour and delivery with at least one other midwife present. It is rare for them to attend births by themselves, with the possible exception of emergency situations when another midwife or birth attendant cannot be present. The philosophy of the Freemont Birth Collective (1977, 20) is clear: two midwives are ordinarily present for births, sometimes a third, but never one. There are instances in Canada where a midwife attends a precipitate labour and delivery by herself. These appear to be very much the exception. Senior community midwives explained that, where possible, they are accompanied by other midwives. The sole responsibility for managing a birth alone is onerous, and there is a commonsense basis to this. Midwives may be faced with emergency situations that require the judgment and skills of two attendants. One community midwife recalled an incident where a home birth became dangerous for mother and the newborn child:

Probably the highest stress of any year in my practice was handling all the responsibility at births for about a year ... it's a huge disadvantage, there is no advantage as far as I am concerned. It's really high stress. And it's really important to have a second opinion, especially if you are emotionally involved and often you have an attachment to the woman. It is helpful to have someone present who doesn't have that rapport and who can look at it more objectively. The turning point for me was when I did a birth alone (in an area where a hospital was not at hand). The woman had a precipitate labour, one hour start to finish for her first birth, which runs a lot of risk for the mother and the baby. The baby didn't breathe and the mother had a massive post-partum haemorrhage. There was a real sense of having only two hands

... the father completely flipped out and left the room. It was managed by giving the mother an injection to stop the bleeding with one hand, and using the other hand to stimulate the baby ... That was the last time I did a birth alone.

Another British Columbia midwife agreed with the wisdom of a shared practice, with at least two midwives attending a home birth: "I always work in a team, unless the birth happens so quickly that the back-up midwife doesen't have time to get there. I have done one or two births under those circumstances, but it is the exception. It isn't planned that way. We always work as a team." This arrangment allows for collegiality, and if midwives work in small groups – for example, four midwives in rotation – they can be spared the around-the-clock demands associated with solo practice (see Benoit 1991).

Community midwives also maintain contacts with general practitioners. This may involve referrals of the midwife's clients to a physician for a check-up; in other cases the contacts are more direct. "The back-up physician for one birth had been at the home, as a friend only, and had been completely informed about the care of this client. The physician knew an hour before we arrived that [this client] would be transferred from home to hospital. The physician called in a specialist that we knew would not be hostile: this specialist likes women and is cooperative with us ... I knew there would be no repercussions against any of us because the whole team had been in on it."

Collaboration between general practitioners and obstetricians and the community midwives indicates that midwifery is not entirely an oppositional movement, and that some medical personnel are sympathetic to the midwives' efforts to re-establish more autonomous midwifery services. One practising midwife recognized that few physicians can afford to support community midwives openly: "There are a few sympathetic physicians in B.C. Some are totally committed to supporting midwives, and will not be pressured out of it. There are physicians who will no longer collaborate with midwives if they face political pressure. These physicians are at the bottom of the list to work with. They aren't committed to home birth or autonomous midwifery, and they really don't believe in a woman's power to give birth. They are quite uptight about this, and like to screen out women seeking home births for *any* risk factor, however slight."

The point remains that physicians who are active with midwives may face sanctions from the College of Physicians and Surgeons. Attending home births is strongly discouraged for physicians, as is collaboration with midwifery initiatives such as the now-disbanded midwifery school. Dr. Marsden Wagner (see *Midwifery and the Law* 1991) of the World Health Organization puts this situation into perspective: "There are physicians in Canada who have the courage and vision to support midwives. They have been punished by their peers. In some cases, physicians have lost their hospital privileges. That's a disaster for a physician."

Caseload

The available literature on lay midwives indicates that caseloads are not particularly high, perhaps because of the organization of lay midwifery practice relative to more formalized practices of obstetricians and general practitioners. A midwifery practice shared by two midwives in a rural area of Montana ranged between twenty and thirty women (Sutley 1982, 80–1). Community midwives in British Columbia generally report that they have more demand for their services than they can provide. It is now fairly common for a community midwife to attend between two and four births monthly. This caseload allows a sufficient monthly income for midwives. It also is a manageable number, since the midwives' time must be allocated to prenatal visits, postnatal check-ups, and time with their own families (most community midwives have children), and meetings and formal instruction. Barrington (1985, 14) found that the contemporary community midwife in Canada plays many roles: "She is a domestic helper, a community worker, and a feminist health activist. Chances are, she is also someone's mother and someone's sweetheart. A midwife doesn't get much sleep!"

Community midwives interviewed by me confirmed that their work was very demanding. They were usually on call for their clients; care for their children was not always at hand if they were called to a birth; and financial pressures added to their stress. It is noteworthy, however, that a number of these midwives have since restricted their caseloads and made arrangements for child care and some additional time for themselves. One midwife spoke of wearing out her welcome, and having to be more resourceful: "I used to rely on friends, but I am doing more births now. I have to really organize the babysitting. I have regular childcare for my youngest child, and after-school care for my oldest. Otherwise, your friendship wears thin with people … If we were in a tighter community where there was more support, then we probably could exchange goods for services and could rely more on our friends. It just makes it so much easier to do prenatal and postnatal visits without the kids if you have a regular set-up."

While this midwife continues to practise in 1993, many other midwives have discontinued practice. Only a handful of the midwives interviewed in 1983–85 now attend home births. This pattern of leaving independent practice as a midwife has become the norm, even for midwives who are now licensed midwives (through the British Columbia School of Midwifery, and accredited in Washington state).

Fees and Payment: "Eggs for a Year"

In the early days of community midwifery, some midwives accepted payment "in kind" in lieu of cash payment (Campbell 1947, 45–7; Klein 1980). In a discussion with a senior community midwife in 1987, she mentioned that she had been given "eggs for a year" after attending a birth in the Kootenay region of British Columbia. An important change has been a clear trend toward more standardized cash payments. One midwife commented that she could no longer afford the altruism of attending births without a clearly specified fee: "Money is not one of my strong points. That was something I have had to deal with. I went through a thing where I had given birth to my first child and had a heavy experience. I felt really grateful to the midwives who attended me. I heard Ina May Gaskin [author of *Spiritual Midwifery* and a founder of The Farm in Tennessee] talking about how birthing should be free, so I decided to exchange goods for services and accept donations. It was something I negotiated with the client and felt really relaxed about. At the time, I was relying on my husband to support me. Since then, my marital status changed, and I have had to become more independent. That meant becoming really clear with myself in how I deal with money, and ensuring that I have a certain amount of work ... What I do now is to find out from other midwives what they are charging, and I charge the same fee."

The spiritual inclination of the 1970s and 1980s has shifted toward a more businesslike stance on the part of some community midwives. The days when a midwife took the bus to a birth or hitchhiked (because she could not afford a car) have passed. One community midwife in British Columbia charged $400 in 1983 for prenatal and postnatal care, labour, and delivery (Padmore 1983, A7). Within limits, this fee may be negotiated by clients of some midwives: "In 1985, my fee for prenatal care, attending the birth, and postpartum care is $600. Often, that will slide down a bit for people who have a low income, but usually not too much. I don't pay fees for a back-up midwife, because I have a partner and we trade births. Many midwives pay the back-up midwife $100 for assisting at a birth. The man I live with also has an income, so we have a combined income. The fees have increased over the years. Now, I have fewer births to attend, and clients are almost guaranteed access to me, 24 hours a day, seven days a week. On average, I attend four births a month. In contrast, I have a friend who practices midwifery in Washington State. Her prenatal visits are probably half the time of mine because she has a busy clinic. Her fee is $900 u.s. And that seems about right."

In the mid-1980s, midwives reported charging approximately $600 for their work, including prenatal and post-partum care, as well as birth attendance. Community midwives may enjoy tax advantages, since they are currently self-employed. Supplies, transportation costs, and costs of electricity, telephone, and office space can sometimes be deducted as employment expenses from taxable income. Nevertheless, midwives rarely make much of a living compared to other health professionals, and many British Columbia midwives have ceased practice in favour of more established work in nursing and public health.

Supplies

Community midwives differ from institutionally based caregivers with respect to access to medical supplies and equipment, including oxygen, intravenous equipment, and drugs. The establishment of professional medical and nursing schools and practices has been accompanied by a degree of control over birthing supplies as well as technical knowledge and practice. Community midwives in British Columbia have access to surgical gloves and scissors, oxygen, and pitocin. It has been observed that practising midwives in British Columbia have fewer difficulties obtaining such supplies than midwives in the United States. One community midwife relied on oxygen supplies, a fetal monitor, and (unspecified) drugs in her practice (Brook 1980, 6). Community midwives in North America can also avail themselves of a variety of technological aids, including telephone answering machines, pagers, and answering services.

Home Births by Province and Year

The records used for the documentary analysis were drawn primarily from community midwives who were active in British Columbia, Ontario, and Saskatchewan. There seems to be a lower incidence of home births in Saskatchewan in comparison with British Columbia, Ontario, and Alberta. One source indicated that there were approx-

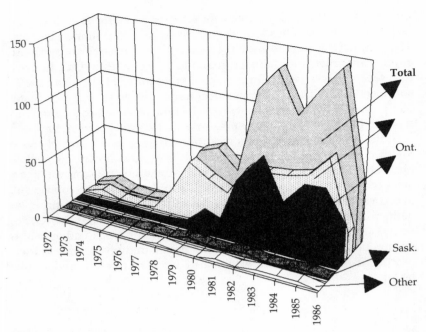

Figure 2
Home Births by Year and Province

imately four home births per month in Saskatoon (Devine 1981, 6).
Until such time as a nationwide system of registration is in place, it
is impossible to determine exact variations in the percentages of
women electing home births. A few home birth records from Manitoba, New Brunswick, California, and Washington state are also
included. These births were attended by Canadian midwives, and
included with the bulk of births occurring in Canada. The entire
sample of records spans the period between 1972 and 1986, with
most records concentrated in the 1980s. Because of incomplete
records, some information, such as the exact year of birth, was not
always recorded by the midwife. Figure 2 outlines the profile of birth
records by year and province.

The difficulty in obtaining records from 1972 to 1977 is apparent
in figure 2. A number of the midwives who were active with a
birthing centre in Vancouver and in attending births have since
moved out of province. Moreover, record-keeping for many midwife-
assisted births in this period was not extensive. This stands in some
contrast to the current emphasis on careful charting of prenatal and
postnatal developments, as well as labour and delivery. Nevertheless,

most births analysed in this chapter occurred between 1978 and
1986, and primarily in British Columbia and Ontario. More recent
reports on home births in Europe, Australia, and Canada are discussed later in the chapter.

Clients

The clients of community midwives vary considerably within British
Columbia. There has certainly been a stronghold of New Age philosophy in the Kootenays, where alternative lifestyles have taken root,
including adaptation of Navajo rituals and traditional healing (Barrington 1985). Dissatisfaction with standard maternity services was
often noted on the prenatal records of home birth clients. The following passage is excerpted from a birth record I reviewed. The
mother had written a letter to her baby, to be read when the child is
older: "I went to a doctor who left me feeling birth care with her
would be like being an object on an assembly line: a woman went
to the hospital when in labour, could continue without intervention
if she performed to the doctor's specifications. Any beliefs I had about
the benefits of a calm, relaxed delivery seemed to be in the hands
of fate. The doctor was too busy to be concerned about such beliefs."

Community midwives expect that their clients will take precautions against poor nutrition and other factors that might pose problems for the fetus or mother. Midwives acknowledge that their clients
are generally health-conscious. One midwife in British Columbia who
had attended hundreds of home births stated: "I have only screened
out one woman for alcohol and drug abuse. The average woman who
comes to me does not have that kind of lifestyle."

Midwives may provide a structure of expectations for women interested in midwife attendance. The following statement of the parents'
role and responsibility is part of an "Informed Choice Agreement"
prepared by two senior community midwives in British Columbia.

We request that the mothers we are involved with be responsible about the
health of themselves and their babies, follow a balanced diet, receive good
prenatal care and get adequate sleep and exercise. We also request that the
couple acquire knowledge and skills necessary for labour and birth and
relaxation, either through completion of prenatal classes, or a sufficient program of self education. A midwife's care is individualized according to the
clients she serves. It is important for you to make her aware of your expectations. In order for us to be effective as caregivers, we require that parents
keep us well-informed as to problems or situations which may affect their
care.

This sense of clients' responsibility is connected with the understanding that not all pregnancies will be carried to term successfully.
Noble (1983, 15) puts this well: "Pessimists may comment that one
should not aspire to natural childbirth in case complications develop.
This is like saying one shouldn't bond with the baby in case it dies,
or one shouldn't fall in love in case one gets hurt. Such timidity and
antilife sentiments lead to self-fulfilling prophecies and deny the
human potential to respond to the unexpected."

The natural childbirth "style" is often captured in the mother's
intention to breast-feed. Of the women attempting to deliver at home,
99.5 per cent intended to initiate breast-feeding. This percentage even
exceeds the 93 per cent figure of breast-feeding among members of
a Parents' Choice sample – that is, women inclined to breast-feed
their infants on discharge from hospital. Other comparison groups
in a Vancouver-based study did not rely as extensively on breast-
feeding. The percentage of women who initiated breast-feeding, by
ethnicity, was as follows: English-Canadian (79 per cent), East Indian
(59 per cent), Italian (50 per cent), Greek (47 per cent), and Chinese
(31 per cent) (see Bradley et al. 1978, 18–19). A study of 123 Malaysian
women found that 75 per cent breast-fed their babies, 22 per cent
combined breast-feeding with bottle-feeding, and only 3 per cent
used formula milk exclusively (Laderman 1983, 84). For virtually all
women in the home birth sample, breast-feeding was seen as clearly
advantageous to mother and infant (see Minchin 1985; Riddell 1992).
Midwives I spoke with encouraged mothers to breast-feed, and were
aware of cultural factors that might discourage women from initiating
or continuing with breast-feeding (see also Hefti 1992; Hewat 1992,
89).

The ages of women attempting home births ranged between 17
and 42 years. The median age of women in the sample was 28 years.
Figure 3 indicates that while births in British Columbia closely parallel
trends across Canada, the home birth sample comprised fewer
younger women (teenagers) and proportionately more women in
their thirties and forties.

Other midwives practising in Alberta report a similar profile of
clients' ages. Their ages ranged from 20 to 42, with an average age
of 28.3 years (Walker et al. 1986). The average age for women (having
live births) in Canada in 1985 was 27.3 years; the median age was
27.1 years (Statistics Canada 1986, 17). Two age groupings that some
regard as high-risk – in terms of statistical risk of birth complications
– were underrepresented. Only a few teenagers attempted a home
birth, and there were few women over 35 in the home birth sample.

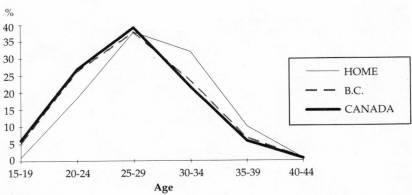

Figure 3
Ages of Home Birth Clients and Women Giving Birth in Canada and British Columbia
Sources: home birth records and Statistics Canada, *Births and Deaths: Vital Statistics 1985,*
November 1986 (Ottawa: Supply and Services Canada) 6–7.

It is important to note that this designation of women over 35 as high-risk has not been upheld by more recent studies.

*Gravida and Parity (Pregnancies and Births)
of Clients*

The number of pregnancies and the number of previous births are two significant variables in establishing a client profile for community midwifery. "Gravida" refers to the number of times a woman has been pregnant, including her pregnancy at the time she is seen by the midwife. "Parity" indicates the number of times she has given birth.

A minority of the sample (22.2 per cent) had previously given birth at home. Most of these women had just one previous home birth (n = 156), twenty-one had two previous home births, and one Mennonite woman had seven previous home births (see also Barrington 1985, 93–100). Approximately one-third of these attempts at home births were made by women who had not given birth previously; about one-third of the sample had had one previous birth.

Income and Occupation of Clients

The variables of income and occupation have been linked with birth outcomes in previous studies of health care. As noted in chapter

Table 1
Gravida and Parity of Home Birth Clients

| | Gravida | | Parity | |
	N	%	N	%
None	na*	na	411	40.9
One	220	22.1	369	36.7
Two	318	31.9	162	16.1
Three	247	24.8	42	4.1
Four	123	12.4	16	1.6
Five	50	5.0	3	0.3
Six	25	2.5	2	0.2
Seven	7	0.7	0	0.0
Eight	1	0.1	0	0.0
Nine	2	0.2	0	0.0
10+	3	0.3	1	0.1
Total	996	100.0	1,006	100.0

Source: home birth records.

* The minimum gravida for this sample is 1. This measure includes the current pregnancy at the time of contact with the midwife.

three, there seems to be a positive correlation between greater income and higher status occupation, and lowered rates of infant mortality.

Community midwives did not usually indicate income of their clients and spouses, although one Ontario midwife tended to record these incomes, along with occupation. What is presented below, then, is a partial profile of couples attempting home birth. It serves, however, as an indicator of the diversity of occupations held by these people. My impression is that fewer lower-income people are evident in the home birth sample in recent years. Community midwives did not usually indicate the income of their clients and the clients' spouses, although one Ontario midwife often recorded these incomes, along with occupations. Table 2 indicates that there is considerable variation in reported family incomes for this sub-sample of women seeking home births.

There is considerable variation in the occupations of the home birth clients and their spouses. There were 54 homemakers listed among the women attempting home birth. Sixteen women were listed as unemployed. There were 10 nurses in the sample. The majority of women (29 of 182 listed) were working in clerical or secretarial positions. There was also a great range in occupations among the spouses of the women attempting home birth; artists and salespersons were the two most frequent categories. A full profile of occupations is

Table 2
Family Income: Home Birth Clients

Gross income	N	%
$10,000–$14,999	4	8.7
$15,000–$19,999	5	10.8
$20,000–$24,999	6	13.1
$25,000–$29,999	9	19.5
$30,000–$34,999	9	19.5
$35,000–$39,999	5	10.9
$40,000 +	8	17.5
Total	46	100.0

Source: home birth records (Ontario sample).

impossible, since most midwives did not indicate clients' occupations on their records. It appears that the home birth alternative is attractive to a fairly broad cross-section of people, and certainly not to a small range of occupations or incomes. Linda Knox, a senior community midwife and president of the Midwives Association of British Columbia, described her clientele as follows: "We have a wide range of backgrounds, including professionals. We have doctors, nurses, lawyers, police officers, upper-middle-class people ... It's important to get away from the picture of the 'lunatic fringe,' which is a statement that a lot of people opposed to midwifery use ... We get people who are well-educated, who have researched the issues around childbirth thoughtfully, before coming to the conclusion that this is what they want: a midwife to look after them, no matter what their place of birth is ... we get a lot of people who are into alternative and more natural things, but the bulk of my clientele are older people ... who have given a lot of thought to their choices" (Interview transcript, *Midwifery and the Law* 1991).

Previous Caesarean Section

There is a continuing debate over the advisability of attempted home births for women attempting a vaginal birth after caesarean (VBAC). The dictum, "Once a caesarean, always a caesarean" has been challenged by research findings that rupture of the uterine scar occurs in a small minority (0.005 to 1.0 per cent) of attempted vaginal deliveries after a caesarean delivery. It is revealing that the Society of Obstetricians and Gynecologists of Canada recently supported a motion favouring VBAC trials of labour (editorial 1986, 62–3). While there is sympathy among many community midwives for women

Table 3
Previous Caesarean Section

	N	%
No births*	252	32.9
No previous C-section	496	64.8
Previous C-section	18	2.3
Total	766	100.0

Source: home birth records.
* This indicates the number of women who had not given birth previously and therefore could not have had a previous caesarean section.

Table 4
Home Birth Clients' Diets

Diet	N	%
Meat	465	70.6
Vegetarian	156	23.7
Seafood	38	5.8
Total	659	100.1

Source: home birth records.

wishing to attempt a vbac at home, many community midwives regard this as a clear contraindication to a home birth: only 3.7 per cent of the birthing clients in this sample attempted a vbac. If the clients who had not given birth previously are excluded, about 5 per cent of the remainder were attempting birth at home after a caesarean section.

Diet and Alcohol Intake

A stereotypical interpretation of midwives' clients is that they are countercultural, and often espouse a vegetarian philosophy. The birth records suggested a more cosmopolitan orientation regarding diet. In fact, the midwives' documents indicated that while a substantial minority of home birth clients were vegetarian (23.7 per cent), over two-thirds included meat in their regular diet.

Heavy alcohol intake during pregnancy may harm unborn children. Fetal alcohol syndrome (fas) refers to fetal malformations such as dysfunctions of fine motor functions, slower weight gain and linear growth, smaller head circumference, and mental retardation. The

Table 5
Home Birth Clients' Alcohol Use during Pregnancy

	N	%
None	355	60.9
Occasional	20	37.7
Daily	8	1.4
Total	583	100.0

Source: home birth records.

Table 6
Smoking among Home Birth Clients

	N	%
Never	560	86.6
Occasionally	16	2.5
Daily	71	10.9
Total	647	100.0

Source: home birth records.

effects of FAS tend to persist after birth (Jensen, Bensen, and Bobak 1979, 809–12; Little and Pytkowics 1978).

According to midwives' birth records, home birth clients were moderate in their alcohol intake, if they consumed alcohol at all during pregnancy. This moderation, combined with the very high percentage of mothers intending to breast-feed and the relatively low percentage of daily smokers, supports the notion that these women tend to follow some standard advice directed toward pregnant mothers and to be responsible in preparing for birth. Only a small percentage of the midwives' clients were daily smokers (see table 6).

This minority of daily smokers very likely reflects a "self-screening" process whereby women interested in a home birth are in general conscious of the risks associated with daily smoking. Midwives are often reluctant to attend women who smoke. Kitzinger (1991, 45) suggests that "many midwives in the USA and Canada will not accept home birth clients who smoke during pregnancy, because of the associated risks." Community midwives are likely to encourage clients to abstain from smoking or to reduce smoking, citing the known risks. This said, not all midwives would categorically screen out clients who smoked. There was a tendency to interpret the smoking in terms of the woman's health and circumstances. A community midwife offered her approach: "I don't automatically screen out a smoker. I tend to base my assessment on how and why they are smoking, and how it affects their nutrition and general health. Some people smoke and are relaxed and enjoy it; other people smoke and are extremely nervous and don't eat well. The person who is a nervous smoker I would not do a home birth for. But someone who smoked, and it was a relaxing, enjoyable thing, and her baby was growing normally and she was eating normally, then I would help deliver the baby at home."

Approximately 80 per cent of the clients reported not using drugs other than alcohol or cigarettes. The most commonly used of these other drugs was marijuana (13.9 per cent), followed by painkillers (3.2 per cent) and insulin for diabetes (0.3 per cent).

Prenatal Visits

Community midwives and midwives working in hospital-based demonstration projects (see Carty et al. 1984) emphasize continuity of care throughout pregnancy. Knowing the client well is part of sound midwifery practice, just as the client's comfort with the midwife is seen as crucial to the best possible delivery. This was evident in the home birth records. Of 466 birth records in which the exact number of visits by the midwife were recorded, only a few cases with no visits or three or fewer visits by the midwife were found. The median number of visits was five, and over a quarter of the women were seen on seven or more occasions. Figure 4 sets out the frequency of prenatal visits as noted on the birth records.

It should be kept in mind that most women also had visits with general practitioners or obstetricians in addition to visits from their midwife (or midwives). Therefore, the statistics presented above do not represent all prenatal visits or consultations for the home birth clients. It is important to note, however, that many visits from midwives lasted an hour or more, sometimes substantially longer. This allowed midwives to build a rapport with clients, and avoided the feeling of being "rushed" sometimes associated with prenatal visits with physicians.

Midwifery Practice and the Course of Labour

Midwives usually claim that their training allows them to minimize interventions during labour and delivery. The available studies from Canada, including updated statistics from community midwives in Alberta (see Hanley 1993, 16), suggest that surgical interventions are

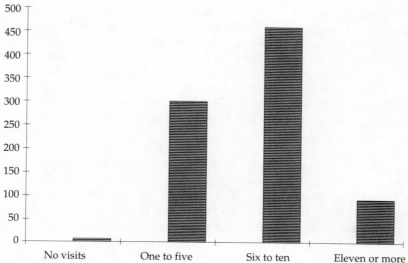

Figure 4
Prenatal Visits by Community Midwives

reduced dramatically for home birth clients. Moreover, measures of morbidity (injury) are also appreciably lower. In my study it was clear that community midwives did not routinely rupture their clients' membranes artificially. Midwives were sparing in the use of oxytocin to induce or augment labour (or expedite delivery of the placenta after birth), and in reliance on painkillers during childbirth. Immobilization of women in labour was also discouraged. Midwives encourage women to move about and to bathe during labour. Furthermore, in keeping with the premise that birth is a personal process, women were encouraged to use delivery positions other than the lithotomy position if they wished (Burtch 1987a, 1988). The following section provides a profile of interventions and techniques associated with the sample of attempted home births.

Rupture of Membranes

A key premise of the community midwives is that by respecting the normal course of labour they provide a service to their clients, and that this protects the unborn child. One measure of their practices is the rupture of the woman's membranes, releasing the amniotic fluid. The great majority of women attempting home birth experienced spontaneous rupture of membranes. Artificial rupture of membranes (ARM) may be employed to induce labour, or more commonly as a procedure when the amniotic sac is bulging and ready to burst. According to 1980–81 data, ARM occurred in 8.6 per cent of all hospital births in Canada (Statistics Canada 1984, 34). In discussing the increased incidence of artificial rupture (in the attempted home birth sample) with several community midwives, they expressed surprise that ARM occurred in about 15 per cent of the sample. Walker et al. (1986) reported ARM in 15.6 per cent of the births they attended between 1980 and 1985. It may be that ARM is used to induce labour, or because a number of women about to give birth at home had intact amniotic sacs just prior to delivery and the sac had to be ruptured to permit delivery of the baby. The national rate of ARM may be lower, since all women giving birth are included. Table 7 indicates that approximately four-fifths of women planning home births had their membranes rupture spontaneously. About 15 per cent had their membranes ruptured artificially at home.

Meconium Staining

The presence of meconium (feces expelled by the infant) in amniotic fluid may indicate fetal distress. All obstetrical and midwifery source-books recommend careful monitoring of the infant's heartbeat during labour if meconium is observed, with special attention to abnormal heartbeats (decelerations or accelerations). Meconium is not, however, an automatic indication of fetal distress. It is customary for the newborn infant to be suctioned with a DeLee catheter to remove meconium or mucus that may endanger the infant's respiratory system (Davis 1981, 104). It is significant that over one-tenth of these attempted home births involved some meconium show (see table 8). It is not always clear from the home birth records what procedures were taken to protect against fetal distress.

Oxytocin

The critique of obstetrical management of childbirth rests in part on what is seen as the unwarranted and routine use of drugs to influence the natural course of labour. The use of oxytocin to induce labour, to augment contractions, or as a routine procedure to assist delivery of the placenta is one case in point. The norm in attempted home deliveries was to avoid the use of oxytocin, although it is more prominent in the third stage of labour (between the birth of the child and expulsion of the placenta). As table 9 indicates, oxytocin was not used for nearly 82 per cent of the sample; it was used for 15 per cent of the women following the birth.

Table 7
Rupture of Membranes in Attempted Home Births

	N	%
Spontaneous	659	80.4
Artificial (home)	124	15.1
Artificial (hospital)	21	2.6
Born in caul	9	1.1
Trailing membranes	7	0.8
Total	820	100.0

Source: home birth records.

Table 8
Meconium in Waters

	N	%
Clear waters	610	83.7
Old meconium	13	1.8
Fresh meconium	30	4.1
Unspecified	76	10.4
Total	729	100.0

Source: home birth records.

Anaesthesia and Analgesia

Anaesthesia was not used in home births: epidurals and general anaesthetics are administered only in hospitals. Emotional support was often provided by the midwives and spouses during painful contractions. Other forms of pain relief included warm baths, massage, and ice packs. Again, this raises the issue of the community of women and how this level of support may reduce the conventional use of anaesthesia and drugs for pain relief. Certainly there have been statements concerning the reliance on technological solutions to birth events, particularly on the degree to which a technological approach to birthing may increase women's fear of labour and promote more instrumental deliveries and the use of pain relief, among other things. Close to 96 per cent of women attempting to give birth at home did not receive anaesthesia; it was used for women transferred to hospital, where an epidural or general anaesthesia might be used (see table 10).

Immobilization of women during labour and delivery has been challenged by some birth attendants and researchers. Walking during

Table 9
Use of Oxytocin in Attempted Home Births

	N	%
No oxytocin given	606	81.8
To induce labour	7	0.9
To augment labour	12	1.6
Post-partum (bleed)	109	14.7
Delivery of placenta	7	0.9
Total	741	99.9

Source: home birth records.

labour is thought to be beneficial for both the mother and the fetus. The duration of labour may be shortened, and blood supply to the fetus may be increased if the mother is not restricted to the lithotomy position. Table 11 shows that 56 per cent of women in the home birth sample walked at some point in their labours. This may be an under-estimate, as not all records would record whether or not the woman was moving about during the labour. Records indicated that some women who intended to walk about did not do so because they were experiencing rapid, strong contractions. Others may simply have been more comfortable in a supine position.

Place of Delivery

Community midwives in Canada have made home birth their primary work, often supplemented with more conventional work, such as labour support for women in hospital. Birthing at home remains very controversial. Some view home birth as a perfectly healthy option for women. Michel Odent (1986, 132) has argued for a stronger appreciation of the benefits of birthing in "a familiar and feminine environment." Attempts to discredit home birth rest not simply on sober science, but on a lack of good will on the part of professionals seeking control in a technologically oriented society: "The subtlest way to discredit home births is to make it as dangerous as possible. It is made dangerous partly by creating an atmosphere of guilt. When a woman dares to think of having a home birth, the first thing she is asked is what she would do if there were complications. Professionals never think that it might be easier if women did not have to leave a familiar place" (Odent 1986, 133).

Categorical opposition to home births is commonplace within the North American medical profession and in many other associations.

Table 10
Anaesthesia in Attempted Home Births

	N	%
No anaesthesia	767	95.6
Epidural only	31	3.9
General only	3	0.4
Epidural and general	1	0.1
Total	802	100.0

Source: home birth records.

Table 11
Walking during Labour

	N	%
Walking	365	56.6
Not walking	280	43.4
Total	645	100.0

Source: home birth records.

Home births are seen not as inherently risky – some opponents concede that many if not most births will proceed well at home – but as hazardous, since complications of birth cannot be predicted with accuracy. The dictum is: "It is much easier to make a hospital birth homely than to make a home birth safe" (Beischer and Mackay 1986, 340). The authors add that complications such as neonatal distress, post-partum haemorrhage, and other potentially serious probems "can never be anticipated with certainty." A number of published studies of home birth demonstrate that most births can be completed successfully at home. A report by midwives practising in Alberta indicated that 7.3 per cent (n = 34) of women seeking a home birth were transferred to hospital and 1.7 per cent of home-born babies were transferred to hospital. Walker et al. (1986, 6) reported that babies were transferred for various problems: meconium aspiration, congenital heart abnormality, fever, spinal abnormalities, respiratory difficulties, and aspiration pneumonia.

Figure 5 indicates that approximately 86 per cent of mothers in the attempted home birth sample delivered at home. It appears that only 8 of these 885 women gave birth at the midwife's home or the home of a friend or relative. There was one case of a mother giving birth

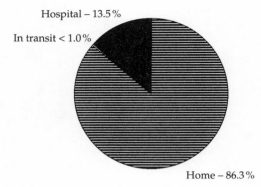

Figure 5
Place of Delivery

in a vehicle during a transfer to hospital. Over 13 per cent of mothers gave birth in hospital after transferring from home.

The commonplace emphasis on complications requiring transfer of home birth clients might be turned on its head. Very little attention is paid in the media to stillbirths in hospital. Of 43,911 live births in British Columbia in 1985, there were 193 stillbirths (of infants over 28 weeks' gestation). This converts to a rate of 4.4 stillbirths per 1,000 live births and specified fetal deaths (Statistics Canada 1986, 4–5). In contrast, stillbirths at home garner considerable media attention and are more likely to be followed by criminal charges against the birth attendants. It is clear, however, that congenital problems that cause the death of an infant are unlikely to result in criminal prosecution of birth attendants whether they are physicians or midwives, in hospital or at home. Linda Knox put the media focus in context: "You have to have a story before the media is involved. Unfortunately, they're quick to pick up on the negatives ... we don't read about the numerous infant deaths in hospitals over a year, but if there is one infant death out of hospital, or with a midwife involved, it's sensational news. There are hundreds of successful deliveries by midwives that aren't written about" (*Midwifery and the Law* 1991).

The next chapter provides more detail on the legal entanglements midwives have faced in Canada and elsewhere. At this juncture, however, it is important to note that the midwives I interviewed emphasized their vulnerability to criminal charges. Physicians and nurses practising in hospitals are shielded from criminal prosecution in practice, while midwives could face prosecution in spite of their record of attending births or even the merits of the case. This gap between formal equality before the law and patterns of prosecuting midwives has often been highlighted in jurisdictions where mid-wives have an illegal or alegal (unclear) status.

Delivery Positions

The importance of matching birth management with the needs of the mother is clearly reflected in the variety of birthing positions adopted by women giving birth. The conventional position for spontaneous vaginal delivery and forceps delivery is the lithotomy position: the woman lies on her back, with flexed knees, and her abducted (drawn away from the mid-body) thighs drawn toward her chest (Jensen et al. 1979, 952). The conventional use of the lithotomy position in hospital deliveries has been criticized for prolonging labour since it does not utilize gravitational force, among other things. Enkin and his associates (1989, 187–8) question the usefulness of encouraging mothers to remain supine during labour. They suggest that "the supine position can adversely affect both the condition of the fetus and the progression of labour, by interference with the uterine blood supply and by compromising the efficiency of the uterine contractions. Frequent changes of maternal position may be a way of avoiding the adverse effects of fetal and maternal outcome."

Attempts by physicians to control delivery positions have prompted protest demonstrations, most notably at the Royal Free Hospital in Hampstead, England in 1982. There, the introduction of active delivery positions, such as delivering in an upright position, had been followed by measures to discourage any position other than on one's back. A protest rally was organized by the National Childbirth Trust. (For an account of this protest, see CSP editors 1982, 64.) Another instance of lobbying for improved maternity and infant services is reported by the Spastics Society (1981).

Results of a recent survey commissioned by the Canadian Medical Association indicate that only 26 per cent of women surveyed had their choices of delivery positions respected by the attending staff (Canadian Press 1987). A more recent survey of nine hundred women in greater Vancouver found that 92 per cent of the respondents agreed that "women should have as much choice as possible during labour and birth, and once the child is born." Specifically, 90 per cent believed that women "should be able to choose the most comfortable birth position for themselves" (Greater Vancouver Regional District 1993, 32).

Community midwives believe that a woman in labour should be able to choose from a variety of positions to find one that is most comfortable for her. Just over four-fifths of the birth records (for

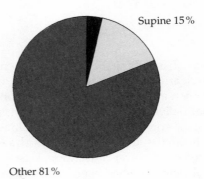

Lithotomy 4%

Supine 15%

Other 81%

Figure 6
Delivery Positions in Attempted Home Births

which delivery position was indicated) mentioned other than lithotomy positions in home births. Women who were transferred to hospital very likely delivered in the lithotomy position or a supine position. It is difficult to establish the exact kinds of position in hospital because midwives' records tended to be weakest if the woman was transferred out of their supervision. Figure 6 compares the delivery positions taken by women attempting a home birth.

A variety of birthing positions were used by women in the home birth sample. The most frequently used position was on hands and knees; a squatting position also was frequently used. A key point is that midwives believe that there is no one delivery position that is suitable for all women. Most records indicated that women used a single delivery position. In about 10 per cent of the births, however, women reportedly used two positions – for example, squatting and then side lying – in delivering their babies.

Type of Delivery

Community midwives as well as nurse-midwives have indicated that through skill and emotional support for birthing women, rates of instrumental deliveries such as caesarean sections and forceps deliveries can be reduced. Indeed, community midwife attendance is accompanied by a dramatic reduction in the rates of instrumental deliveries. Caesarean deliveries accounted for 21.67 per cent of live births in British Columbia in 1991. The rates in Vancouver (21.70 per cent) and greater Victoria (22.77 per cent) closely match the provincial

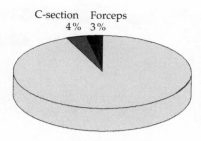

C-section Forceps
4% 3%

Spontaneous Vaginal 93%

Figure 7
Type of Delivery in Attempted Home Births

average (British Columbia 1992, 46). In the United States, the caesarean section rate has increased from 4.5 per cent twenty-five years ago to 24.1 per cent in 1992 (Taffel et al., 1992, cited in Page 1993, 1479). The national rate for caesarean section was 15.9 per cent in 1980–81, compared with a rate of under 5 per cent for the attempted home births (see figure 7 below). Likewise, the percentage of forceps deliveries among the attempted home birth sample (2.9 per cent) is substantially lower than the nationwide rate of approximately 20 per cent (Statistics Canada 1984, 34).

Episiotomies

Community midwives contend that with perineal massage and support and skilful management of birth, most women can deliver babies without episiotomies (surgical enlargement of the vaginal opening). The episiotomy rate in Canada has been estimated at over 80 per cent for primiparas and between 50 and 60 per cent for multiparas (Klein 1993). While data on episiotomies are "best estimates" only, Statistics Canada (1992, 34) reported that 73,253 episiotomies were performed in Canada in 1989–90. The scale of episiotomy is thus striking, especially when scientific studies have challenged the routine use of the procedure (Klein et al., 1992, 1993). These figures may reflect the higher rate of caesarean sections nationwide, for those births do not require episiotomies. Figure 8 depicts the dramatic decrease in episiotomies among attempted home births relative to hospital statistics.

In their review of the available literature on episiotomies, Thacker and Banta (1983) concluded that there is no clear evidence of the benefits of routine use of episiotomies. They added that episiotomies

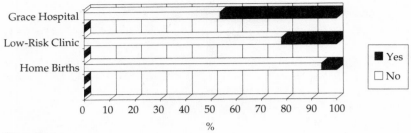

Figure 8
Episiotomy Rates in Home Births, at the Low-Risk Clinic, and at Grace Hospital
Source: home birth records, and Elaine Carty et al., *The Low-Risk Clinic* (1984: 20–1).

are associated with discomfort and pain for women during the post-partum period, and some maternal deaths have been attributed to infections following episiotomy. Midwives argue that the interventionist training of many physicians promotes the routine use of epi-siotomies. Moreover, perineal tears can often be avoided through perineal massage and support of the perineal area during crowning of the infant's head. Deliveries over an intact perineum are most common in the home birth sample. As noted in the previous table, the Low-Risk Clinic clients had a relatively low rate of episiotomy (22 per cent), compared with hospital-wide statistics collected at the Grace Hospital in March 1983.

The following table presents a comparison of perineal tear rates at Grace Hospital, at the Low-Risk Clinic, and among the community midwives. It should be noted that twenty unspecified tears were documented in the home birth records. Since the degree of the tear could not be assessed, they have been included as a separate row in table 12.

Post-Partum Measures

Suctioning of the newborn baby was undertaken in a considerable number of home births in the study. In some cases this is a precautionary measure; in others where the infant is in respiratory distress it may be a life-saving measure. Table 13 shows that suctioning is not routinely undertaken by the community midwives as a group. It can, however, be used as part of the midwives' repertoire, especially if the infant appears to have inhaled meconium or mucus during labour or delivery. Midwives seemed to regard suctioning as a relatively non-invasive procedure, and one that often assisted the newborn and served to check for substances that might obstruct breathing.

Table 12
Perineal Tears

	Home births		Low-risk clinic	
	N	%	N	%
Intact	362	41.8	7	14.3
First degree	308	35.6	20	40.8
Second degree	121	13.9	11	22.4
Third degree	13	1.5	0	0.0
Fourth degree	1	0.1	0	2.0
Unspecified	20	2.3	na	na
Episiotomy	40	4.7	11	22.5
Total	865	99.9	49	100.0

Source: home birth records, Elaine Carty et al., The Low-Risk Clinic (1984: 20–21).

Apgar Scores

The Apgar scoring method was developed in the 1950s by Dr. Virginia Apgar, an American anesthesiologist. The infant's health after delivery is conventionally assessed on five measures – heart rate, respiration, muscle tone, colour, and reflexes – at one minute and five minutes after birth. Thus, a child who is given a maximum rating of two points on each of these five measures would have an Apgar score of ten. A score of zero indicates that the child is stillborn. Intermediate scores indicate some deficits in the child's health at the time the measure is taken. Scores in the lower range can indicate serious difficulties in the newborn's health.

This composite measure of newborn health is usually recorded by community midwives. Table 14 shows the distribution of Apgar scores for infants delivered at home. Apgar scores are generally within the normal range for newborn infants. As table 14 indicates, there is a predictable increase in the Apgar scores over time for most infants. The small number of cases coded for ten minutes after birth (n = 215) occurs because midwives tended to not record Apgar scores at ten minutes unless there was infant distress.

Delivery of Placenta

The third stage of labour comprises the time between the delivery of the baby and the delivery of the placenta. Spontaneous delivery of the placenta occurs when it is expelled without partial (or complete) manual removal, and when oxcytocin is not used to hasten

Table 13
Suctioning Techniques in Attempted Home Births

	N	%
No suctioning	405	53.9
Bulb syringe	103	13.7
De Lee	117	15.6
Unspecified	126	16.8
Total	751	100.0

Source: home birth records.

delivery. Birth records often indicated "controlled cord traction" by the midwife; however, this procedure is classified as a spontaneous delivery provided that oxytocin or manual removal was not used. Table 15 indicates that over 90 per cent of placental removals were unassisted, or "spontaneous."

Delivery of the placenta was assisted in hospital for thirty-one cases (3.8 per cent of all cases). Manual removal of the placenta was undertaken in four cases (0.5 per cent of all cases). Walker et al. (1986, 5) reported that only a small minority (0.7 per cent) of births required manual removal of the placenta.

Neonatal, Perinatal, and Infant Mortality:
A Review

The debate over whether community midwifery is dangerous or desirable is not simply ideological. There have been a number of research studies addressing the issue of safety in planned home deliveries compared with planned hospital deliveries and the nature of the attendants as correlated with birth outcome. Standard measures include perinatal mortality (deaths between 20 weeks' gestation and of neonates between birth and the following six days), neonatal mortality (deaths during the first 28 days after birth), and infant mortality (deaths between birth and the first year of life). In the discussion of the Canadian home birth study that follows, only the first two measures (perinatal and neonatal mortality) are used. The community midwives' records do not cover the full first year of a baby's life. Some exponents of midwifery argue that trained midwifery attendance is associated with better outcomes – lower rates of maternal and infant morbidity and mortality – than physician-managed births. An Illinois physician also concluded that home deliveries, if properly managed, could be safer than hospital deliv-

Table 14
Apgar Scores in Home Births

	1 minute		5 minutes		10 minutes	
	N	%	N	%	N	%
Zero	5	0.6	5	0.6	5	2.3
One	3	0.4	0	0.0	0	0.0
Two	3	0.4	1	0.1	0	0.0
Three	8	0.9	2	0.2	1	0.5
Four	21	2.4	0	0.0	1	0.5
Five	22	2.5	12	1.4	0	0.0
Six	49	5.7	6	0.7	0	0.0
Seven	86	9.9	13	1.5	1	0.5
Eight	207	23.8	40	4.6	3	1.5
Nine	331	38.1	230	26.5	13	6.0
Ten	133	15.3	558	64.4	191	89.0
Total	868	100.0	867	100.0	215	100.0

Source: home birth records.

Table 15
Delivery of Placenta

	N	%
Spontaneous	762	92.5
Assisted	62	7.5
Total	824	100.0

Source: home birth records.

eries. He believed that the home was generally bacteriologically safer, and that physicians assisting at home were more cautious (White 1977, 291–2).

Others have produced mixed findings regarding the home birth issue and the question of qualified attendants. A research team studying neonatal deaths in North Carolina reported that the neonatal mortality rate among the 242,245 babies delivered in hospital was 12 per 1,000 live births. For physicians attending a planned home delivery, there were no infant deaths among the 55 cases recorded. For trained lay midwives attending home deliveries the neontal mortality rate was 4 per 1,000 live births; moreover, the 3 deaths among the 768 babies delivered were related to congenital abnormalities. In one study of home births in North Carolina between 1974 and 1976, Burnett and his associates (1980) found that the rate of infant mortality varied as a function of planning for such births and midwifery attendance. Specifically, planned home deliveries with lay midwives in attendance has a rate of 3 neonatal deaths per 1,000 live births. The corresponding rate for planned home deliveries without lay midwives was 30 per 1,000; for unplanned home deliveries the neonatal death rate increased dramatically to 120 deaths per 1,000 live births (Burnett et al. 1980).

One study of Hutterite midwives used physicians' records and birth certificates for Hutterite children born in Montana between 1961 and 1970. Converse, Buker, and Lee (1973) found that 63 per cent of deliveries of Hutterite children in their sample were attended by indigenous midwives. These Hutterite midwives were not trained in medicine or midwifery. The infant mortality rate for Hutterite children in these communities was not significantly different from that for Hutterite children delivered by physicians or for non-Hutterite Caucasian children delivered by physicians. Nevertheless, the neonatal mortality rate for Hutterite births managed by indigenous midwives was higher than Hutterite births attended by physicians; specifically, 16.4 versus 8.1 deaths per 1,000 live births. Additional problems included the midwives' lack of instruments to monitor fetal and maternal vital signs, infrequent and inadequate prenatal visits, reliance on the lithotomy position, and difficulties associated with managing uterine dystocia, cephalopelvic disproportion, and abnormal presentation of the fetus.

The best evidence, however, is that with proper screening procedures, timely transfer of mothers experiencing complications, and trained attendants, home birth does not result in higher rates of infant or maternal mortality. A large-scale study by Mehl and his associates (1977) in northern California studied 1,146 home births attended by midwives, physicians, or both. They found that birth outcomes and rates of complications compared favourably with average rates in California.

A variety of studies of home birth outcomes in Britain and Holland have been published (Campbell et al. 1979; Klein et al. 1983; Damstra-Wijmenga 1984; for a general review see Tew 1985, 390–4 and Flint 1986, 29–30). All confirm that home birth compares favourably with hospital deliveries in terms of neonatal and perinatal mortality. Home births have also been associated with lower rates of medical intervention in the birthing process.

Marjorie Tew's *Safer Childbirth* (1990) develops an argument against equating improved birth outcomes with physician attendance. Using statistics from Holland – where 36 per cent of births in 1986 occurred at home, and where midwives tend to manage births "according to their own principles" – she found that the perinatal mortality rate (PNMR) was not lowered by hospital-based, physician attendance. Tew (1990, 267) reported that "the PNMR for all births was higher for doctors in hospital (18.9) than for doctors at home (4.5), which was in turn higher than for midwives in hospital (2.1), which was in turn higher than for midwives at home [1.0]." Tew (1990, 270) concludes not only that these findings question the advantages of obstetrical management of birth, "but even that [obstetrical management] actually provokes and adds to the dangers."

A study of 3,400 planned home births in Australia lends weight to these findings. Bastian and Lancaster's (1990) assessment (noted in Kitzinger 1991, 41) revealed that caesarean sections were rare (2.2 per cent), forceps and vacuum extraction deliveries accounted for only 3.1 per cent of births, and episiotomies (20.1 per cent) were substantially less frequent than the national rate of 39.9 per cent. Kitzinger (1991, 41) remarks that some women planning to give birth at home were classified as high-risk. Moreover, "30.8 percent were what doctors called 'untried pelvises,' because they were giving birth for the first time."

A recent review of the debate over place of birth, safety, and morbidity rates underscores the difficulties of establishing cause-and-effect relationships on the basis of existing studies. Campbell and Macfarlane (1987) nevertheless conclude that "there is no evidence to support the claim that the safest policy is for all women to give birth in hospital." The authors note that there is evidence, albeit inconclusive, that morbidity rates are higher for low-risk mothers giving birth in institutions than for other low-risk women giving birth at home. The authors add that "a majority of women who have experienced both home and hospital deliveries prefer to have their babies at home." They caution that this finding may reflect a "disproportionate number" of mothers who chose home birth after an unsatisfactory experience of birth in hospital (Campbell and Macfarlane 1987, 58). While the question whether women electing home birth are a healthier population in general than women delivering in hospital remains unanswered, there is clear support for the safety of home birth in some circumstances. It is important that women be screened for complications, that there be adequate prenatal care, that birth attendants be skilled in domiciliary mangement, and that back-up (emergency) services be in place. Attention has been drawn to ways in which diagnosis of risk, not actual risk, may contribute to increased caesarean section rates (Francome 1986).

With respect to this study, three essential dimensions in infant deaths are employed. First, the accurate measurement of such deaths; second, careful comparisons of time-frames; and finally, attribution

Table 16
Perinatal Mortality (per 1,000 births)

	British Columbia (home deliveries)		British Columbia (provincial)		Canada	
	N	R	N	R	N	R
Perinatal death	3	12.34	na	10.9	na	13.0

Source: home birth records. The B.C. perinatal mortality rate is taken from 1979 data, the Canada-wide rate from 1978 statistics. See Roger Tonkin, 1981.

of responsibility for the deaths. Since reports of infant deaths must be made under the Vital Statistics Act in Canada, difficulty does not usually arise with respect to infants who die at or near term. There are, however, various forms of fetal loss at earlier stages of pregnancy, including planned abortions (therapeutic abortions) and spontaneous abortions (miscarriages)

Two standard measures of fetal and infant death are used in this study. Perinatal mortality measures death of a fetus of 20 or more weeks' gestation or of a neonate between birth and the following six days. Neonatal mortality is a more specific measure, addressing neonatal deaths during the first 28 days after birth. Both measures are expressed as the number of deaths per 1,000 live births. The last dimension will be discussed at greater length after the following measures of mortality. It is important, however, to distinguish between unavoidable infant deaths that may be due to congenital malformations and those that may be attributable to caregivers' negligence. The latter are referred to as iatrogenic (physician-caused) deaths (Illich 1977). As it is used here, the term refers to negligence generally associated with caregivers, whether physicians, nurses, or midwives.

The perinatal mortality rates shown in table 16 were arrived at by dividing the number of stillbirths plus the number of early neonatal deaths (during the first week after birth) by the number of live births and the number of stillbirths, then multiplying the result by 1,000.

The perinatal mortality rate calculated above should be interpreted with caution. It is possible that the rate might have increased if all attempted home births in British Columbia and the other provinces had been analysed. I have not sought access to midwives who were not closely associated with the Midwives Association of British Columbia, nor have I referred to another community midwife who left British Columbia in 1981 after an infant death following an attempted home birth. It is arguable that exclusion of these records may artificially lower the actual mortality rates of midwife-attended attempted home births.

There are other possibilities, however. One community midwife who attended hundreds of births in British Columbia provided a small sampling of records that included a few perinatal deaths, including a stillborn twin. She had not been the primary care midwife for the woman, and was reluctant to deliver twins out of hospital. Nevertheless, she agreed to assist the woman who was about to deliver the babies. The point here is that the sample of attempted home births is missing thousands of births that occurred between 1972 and 1986, and it is not possible to measure precisely the safety of hospital birthing alongside home births. It is generally agreed that existing studies – which are not randomized controlled studies – cannot conclusively establish whether or not home births are safer than hospital or clinic births (Tyson 1988, 39).

A second point is that community midwives did not always select the most healthy clients. There are cases of women who might have been screened out of home birth guidelines who later delivered at home. It should be kept in mind that many women delivering in hospital are healthy, and many have received good prenatal care. Community midwives indicate that perinatal mortality rates are not higher for populations intending to deliver at home. This issue does not necessarily revolve around a dichotomy of community midwifery versus hospital births. Penny Armstrong, an Ontario midwife who has practised midwifery with Amish women, provides a contemporary account of midwifery practice at home and in hospital (see Armstrong and Feldman 1986).

In his study of birth statistics in British Columbia, Tonkin (1981, 18) concluded that "the mortality rate for infants born at home is not markedly different from that of hospital born infants." A report on 465 home births in Alberta between 1980 and 1985 indicated that there were only 3 infant deaths and 1 stillbirth. This converts to a perinatal mortality rate of 8.68 per 1,000 live births (Walker et al. 1986, 1). The measure of neonatal deaths presented in table 17 shows a similarity between domiciliary midwifery outcomes and province-wide and Canada-wide comparisons.

These comparisons appear to support the community midwives' claims that planned home births are not necessarily more dangerous than hospital-based births. These findings are consistent with earlier published reports of low rates of perinatal and neonatal mortality among women seeking home births supervised by trained midwives. The corresponding figure for births managed by midwives on the Summertown Community Farm, Tennessee, a holistic birthing centre,

Table 17
Neonatal Mortality (per 1,000 births)

	British Columbia (home deliveries)		British Columbia (provincial)		Canada	
	N	R	N	R	N	R
Neonatal death	4	4.97	na	6.7	na	8.1

Sources: home birth records, Statistics Canada, Births and Deaths, vol. I (1984).

was 11.1 neonatal deaths per 1,000 live births (Gaskin 1978, 104). Holliday Tyson, in her research into 1,001 home births in Toronto, summarized her findings as follows: 93 per cent of the sample had spontaneous vaginal births; 3.5 per cent had caesarean sections; and 17 per cent of mothers and infants were transferred. Tyson (1988, 40) concludes that her data "show the Toronto home birth population to have a high rate of spontaneous vaginal birth, low rates of surgical interventions, low episiotomy rate, and relatively low rates of perineal lacerations requiring sutures."

Post-Partum Visits

The period following the birth of a child is critically important for mothers and infants. One midwife reported that while she gives attention to various measures of wellbeing of the mother and child, the intimate contact between herself and the client is also important. The midwife explained: "I have a post-partum flow sheet with everything categorized that should be checked. The post-partum care is every day for the first five days, sometimes twice a day depending on the situation. If the birth has been complicated in any way, then I will stay overnight, and usually for the first 18 hours. Every day for the first five days no matter who it is, no matter how normal the birth. That's partly because it takes time to wind down the relationship." She emphasized that the post-partum is not strictly a medical procedure: "Often, the post-partum will have nothing to do with checking what's happening physically, but everyone needs to talk about the birth ... The women really need that because so much is lost to them because they are so inside of themselves, labouring ... it depends, however, since some women don't need to be in such close contact post-partum."

There were exceptions to the norm of visiting, usually due to circumstances outside of the midwives' control. One midwife reported that a client disappeared from the area shortly after the birth (and, incidentally, without paying the midwife for her services). In other cases where the birth took place some distance from the midwife's home, the midwife might stay for a few days after birth. Telephone calls might also be made in lieu of personal visits to the mother's home. There was considerable variation in the number of postnatal visits. Figure 9 shows that ordinarily a midwife made at least three post-partum visits to assess the mother and the newborn.

It may be that midwives did not document all home visits. If this is the case, it underscores the need for improved documentation of practice, including post-partum activities of community midwives. It is my impression that charting of births and midwifery practice has become more thorough since the early to mid-1970s. For example, the Midwives Association of North America (MANA) has devised a comprehensive statistics form (revised 1993) that charts demographic information, the woman's reproductive history, prenatal care, and so forth.

Safe Practice: Guidelines and Peer Review

The issue of infant and maternal safety is central to discussions of childbirth. Feminist critiques of conventional obstetrics often point to reduced freedoms for parturient women, erosion of community contacts, and the substantial power vested in the (predominantly male) medical profession (see Corea 1985; Cox 1991; Treichler 1990). It is also asserted that midwife attendance (at home or in hospital) can be as safe as or safer than physician-managed hospital deliveries. In British Columbia, many community midwives have devised collective standards and peer review procedures to assess what constitutes safe practice. Most practising community midwives are members of the Midwives Association of British Columbia (MABC) with several members founding a separate Midwives Collective.

The 1986 *Guidelines to Midwifery Practice* are taken from the experience of community midwives, the Board of Directors of the MABC, and general lists of contraindications to home birth. The MABC guidelines provide a comprehensive list of procedures for the community midwives. These procedures include initial and ongoing assessments of the client's social and family history, obstetrical and gynecological history, physical examination, and testing for urinalysis, blood pressure, pulse, and the like. The midwife may also refer the client to laboratory specialists for such work as Rh antibodies, hemoglobin, and rubella titre. The schedule for prenatal care is set out as follows: a monthly visit up to the twenty-eighth week of pregnancy; a biweekly visit thereafter until the thirty-sixth week; and weekly visits

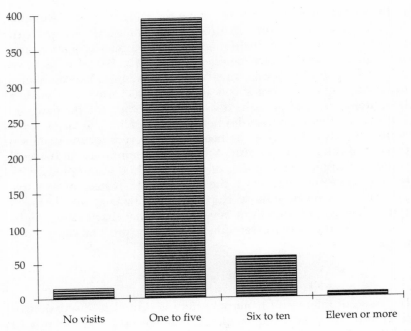

Figure 9
Post-Partum Visits by Community Midwives

from that point until the birth. Measures of blood pressure, weight gain, fetal heart tones, fundal height, and so on should be taken by the midwife. The midwife is expected to maintain accurate records of these visits and to monitor whether these measures are "within normal limits." There is an accompanying list of guidelines that are presented as "definite" indications for a hospital birth. Definite contraindications to a home birth include the following maternal factors: "cardiovascular disease, congenital heart disease, essential hypertension, vascular disease, achondroplasia, drug addiction or abuse, acute psychiatric problems, renal disease, endocrine disorders, thrombosis, emboli, Addison's disease, hypo/hyper thyroid, diabete[s] mellitus, neoplastic disease, immunocomplex disease, history of subarchnoid haemorrhage, TORCH infections, uterine infection, active tuberculosis, and asthma." Midwives disregarding these contraindications may be brought forward for peer review, which is not a formal disciplinary hearing.

Other contraindications to home birth are grouped under two headings. The first heading, "Obstetrical history," includes three or more successive spontaneous abortions, a previous unexplained still-

birth, and previous uterine surgery (which includes a previous caesarean section). The second heading, "Obstetrical Factors in the
Current Pregnancy," includes intrauterine growth retardation, multiple pregnancy (such as twins), confirmed fetal heart abnormalities,
and, inter alia, premature rupture of membranes (before thirty-seven
weeks).

There is also an extensive list of possible indications for a hospital
birth. The midwife is expected to consult with a physician when
such situations occur as smoking during pregnancy, when the mother
is more than 30 minutes away from the nearest hospital, when the
mother is less than 17 or over 40, and when there is abnormal weight
gain.

These guidelines, taken with subsequent guidelines for intrapartum care and postnatal care, appear to be a synthesis of international guidelines for midwifery and local debates over responsible
midwifery practice. The key point here is whether midwives can be
held accountable for ignoring guidelines, especially when some of
them are not very specific. What constitutes "drug addiction or
abuse"? Should the woman be automatically screened out for home
delivery if her membranes rupture at just over thirty-six weeks but
all other factors are well within guidelines?

The interpretation of the rules at present appears less formal,
allowing the midwives some discretion in their work. Midwives are
urged to not attend home births except for singletons; that is, multiple
births should be managed in hospitals. One midwife recalled how
one client, who was intent on a home delivery, had to be referred to
another practitioner:

I had a client who was going to have twins. The bottom line for her, after
all the information, was that she would still choose to birth at home. My
dilemma was, how to support her? In another climate, where midwifery is
legal, there would be a process whereby that woman could still make that
choice, and her caregiver would be protected from the consequences. [The
midwife] would notify her superiors ... she would be able to continue to
care for the woman with some kind of legal protection ... my personal choice
in this case was to say "no," not only because of the legal consequences if
anything was to go wrong, but also because I know what my skills are. I
don't deliver twins; I don't do breeches, which are common in multiple
pregnancies.

Some midwives indicated that they had adopted a more cautious
approach to attending home births: "I don't do VBACS [vaginal birth
after caesarean section] at home now, although I have managed some

VBACs at home over the years. [I may do it] for women who decided at the last moment that they wouldn't go into hospital. I think that VBAC can be done safely at home, but it is something that requires screening ... Politically, it is suicidal for midwives to do it, and I am very committed [to the legalization of autonomous midwifery]. I found there was a lot of pressure if I did a VBAC at home. Once, I was bombarded with telephone calls from physicians who were angry with me for attending a VBAC at home. Also, there is a risk factor. It is a high-stress birth and I am not really relaxed when I am there."

WORLDWIDE, there has been a clear shift to almost complete hospitalization of birth. Once established as a viable alternative to hospital-based obstetrics, the practice of domiciliary obstetrics in Britain, including the "flying squads" staffed by an anaesthetist, an obstetrician, and a midwife in the event of birth complications (da Cruz 1969) has given way to almost universal recourse to hospital obstetrics. It has been reported that approximately 97 per cent of births in Britain take place in hospitals (Kitzinger 1978, 51) and more recent statistics for England and Wales (1991) reveal that only 1.1 per cent of births are home births ("Home Birth Percentages" 1992). In Britain, the delivery of the Prince of Wales at home by Sir John Peel has been followed by the general recommendation by a commission headed by Dr. Peel that all deliveries in Britain occur in hospital (Kitzinger 1978a, vii). The official policy in Britain has thus discouraged domiciliary midwifery. Jean Donnison (1981, 9) remarks, "Despite the lip-service paid by successive Health Ministers to patient choice in the matter of home or hospital delivery under the Health Service (which, incidentally, means at no charge), any woman wanting a home birth on the National Health Service must possess the political skill of a Metternich, the patience of a Griselda and the persistence of a Pankhurst. If she is to succeed, she must begin to fight the Health Service bureaucracy as soon as possible in her pregnancy and be prepared to continue, perhaps for months, in order to overcome the almost insurmountable obstacles put in her way."

There have been a number of initiatives to estabish a more pluralistic maternity and infant care system. It is not at all difficult to establish the borders of debate over the appropriateness of home birth. Some support out-of-hospital birthing clinics and home birth; others decry home births as "the earliest form of child abuse" (Pearse 1977, 1979). Others encourage pregnant women to deliver at home and to lobby for the legal right for childbirth attendants to practise domiciliary obstetrics and midwifery (Bittman and Zalk 1978; Brooks and Bennett 1976; Kitzinger 1978, 1991; Kitzinger and Davis 1978). Clearly, then, the struggle over birth attendance is in large measure a political and ideological debate over power and women's freedom of reproduction. The political and ideological dimensions of this debate are brought forward in the next section, with specific reference to the role of law in regulating birth practices.

Midwifery and the Law

An understanding of the community midwife movement in British Columbia is best located within the broad paradigm of conflict theory within sociology. Childbirth became a battleground between "lay" midwives, doctors, nurses, and scientists. Struggles over childbirth attendance in England reflected longstanding "inter-professional rivalries" (Donnison 1977, 1988). The nature of the conflict is complex, involving not only the economic interests of the established professions and the alternative practitioners, but disagreements among various groupings in the public over safety and standards and the gatekeeping functions of state officials. The conflict approach as applied in the case of midwifery invariably addresses the self-interest of the medical profession in presiding over childbirth and the premise that medical attendance is demonstrably superior to midwifery attendance (Hamowy 1984).

One point worth emphasizing is that the nature of the conflict is not static. Even powerless people can struggle against oppression, occasionally relying on the rule of law to secure their rights (Thompson 1977). This is also true of community midwives, since they reject unfavourable interpretations of their work, continue to practise midwifery, and lobby for the legalization of midwifery. Public education campaigns and media submissions – most notably, letters to newspaper editors – are the more visible lobbying techniques; workshops and educational initiatives, such as the British Columbia School of Midwifery, reflect less visible, collective initiatives to improve community midwifery services. As of 1993, the most successful of these initiatives was a partnership among three post-secondary institutions in Ontario. Laurentian University, McMaster University, and Ryerson Polytechnical University now offer a four-year baccalaureate program in midwifery (Williams 1993).

Other activities within the community midwifery movement include fundraising by means of dances, casinos, and mail solicitation. These activities are usually designed to benefit a group, such as the School of Midwifery, or to defray legal costs associated with coroners' inquests or criminal prosecution following an infant's death. The resources of community midwives are paltry in comparison with the financial resources available to the state and through provincial and national medical associations. Midwives can innovate, however. Nine community midwives began a collective in which education is ongoing and in which each of the members has pledged to contribute up to a thousand dollars in the event that any one member of the collective faces legal costs.

As it evolves, community midwifery in Canada is a hybrid form of midwifery. With ties to a tradition of local self-help and some links with modern New Age spiritual philosophy, a number of practitioners also have formal instruction in nursing and midwifery. Guidelines for midwifery practice have been drafted (and redrafted), and peer review is one mechanism that mirrors a more professional approach to birth attendance by community midwives. The community midwives are not wholly united, however. Some midwives are not affiliated with the MABC, and express serious concerns about the co-option of midwifery as it becomes state-supported. There is disagreement over the appropriateness of attempting home birth without sufficient medical back-up, the availability of emergency services (ambulance transport), whether women who have had a caesarean section should attempt a vaginal birth at home, and so forth.

Community midwifery has faced troubles from without. State measures are taken against community midwives. Criminal prosecution of midwives and other birth attendants has been implemented in British Columbia (and elsewhere), as has prosecution under the provincial Medical Practitioners Act for practising medicine without a licence. The costs incurred in retaining a defence lawyer and the loss of income (if the midwife is forbidden to practice midwifery pending the outcome of a court case), along with the uncertainty of the eventual verdict, reflect some influences of the state on these midwives.

Other measures bear on our theoretical understanding of the state, the professions, and community initiatives. Despite years of lobbying for legal status for midwives and notwithstanding a substantial evaluation literature documenting the benefits of skilled midwifery practice, community midwives remain illegal practitioners under this provincial legislation. They cannot bill under the provincial medical insurance plan, and they lack a substantial defence fund in the event that they are charged with criminal or quasi-criminal offences. Nevertheless, this lack of resources is not always evident when midwives face legal actions. As discussed in chapter five, an Alberta midwife,

Noreen Walker had over $20,000 in her legal defence fund, as well as access to the pro bono services of an Edmonton lawyer.

Paradoxically, community midwives are relatively free to practise and even to advertise their home birth practices, to develop an academic curriculum and practical training, and to transfer women to hospital if a home birth is not successful. This freedom is circumscribed, however, by their complete exclusion from provincial health insurance plans. It is further constrained by the general powers of the medical associations through the state and the reluctance of state officials to further expand medical coverage. The preliminary evidence on the midwifery movement seems best suited to a "relative autonomy" perspective on the state. Liberal democratic states will vary in terms of the degree of their autonomy from civil society. The point remains that the state is not acting simply as an instrument of powerful interests, nor is it promoting the pluralistic principles often linked with liberalism.

In the wake of three coroners' inquests into baby deaths in Ontario, and following years of pressure by the Ontario Midwives' Association (composed of midwives and consumer advocates, among others) and other pro-midwife organizations, midwifery is now legally recognized in Ontario. The Ontario minister of health has proposed direct entry into midwifery (rather than mandatory nursing training in addition to or in place of midwifery training).

The task force on the implementation of midwifery in Ontario recommended a framework that would recognize and regulate midwifery practice. The task force recommended a separate Midwives Act, with the midwife's scope of practice corresponding to the international definition of the midwife. A system of consultations and referrals between midwives and physicians was favoured, although the profession would be self-regulating through a college of midwifery. Home births should be recorded in a central registry to assess mortality and morbidity more systematically. A four-year baccalaureate program was favoured, with a twelve- to eighteen-month program for applicants with nursing qualifications. One point of concern is that some community midwives would be effectively outlawed: the task force report (1987, 19) recommended that "no midwife be permitted to practise except in a practice, service, agency or other health facility approved by the Ministry of Health."

The arguments for legalized midwifery, centring on the safety of home births attended by trained midwives, the so-called soft measures of client satisfaction, and the fundamental democratic principle that the state should not interfere with private decisions of citizens, are quite strong, as are the measures taken to stifle autonomous midwifery practice. The obstacles to the legalization of midwifery in Canadian jurisdictions seem to reflect professional resistance to autonomous midwifery practice and the reluctance of the state to permit community-based, decentralized initiatives at a time when state trajectories are moving toward greater control.

Nevertheless, it must be emphasized that the state in Canada is relatively autonomous, and the degree of autonomy is neither a static nor a permanent feature of the capitalist state. The administration of health is a provincial responsibility, and there have been varying degrees of response from the provinces toward recognizing midwifery in law and public policy. Ontario is in the forefront of legalizing midwifery, and Alberta has made provision for legal midwifery. British Columbia has reviewed a number of submissions proposing direct entry midwifery training and a legal status separate from the nursing and medical professions. In contrast, Quebec midwives have faced serious obstacles, including strong resistance from the medical profession. A recent memo from representatives of the Alliance Québécoise des Sages-Femmes Practiciennes (AQSFP) drew attention to some of these obstacles. Despite the passage in 1990 of a bill that provided for "a five year study of midwifery services within a framework of selected pilot projects," midwives have yet to achieve an established facility for midwifery practice. Moreover, currently they have no voting status on committees established to review these pilot projects, or to assess qualifications for midwifery practice. The authors of the memo protest this failure to implement a more visionary form of midwifery – along the lines followed by the Ontario task force and the Ontario government – and anticipate that midwifery initiatives will be co-opted: "The very real risk here is that midwifery positions in the pilot projects will be filled by midwives, nurses, or doctors who have very little actual experience providing continuous and complete midwifery care on their own responsibility in collaboration with other health care professionals ... The result will at best be a duplication of services and at worst a total mockery in terms of evaluation of competent and appropriate midwifery practice. In any event, an opportunity to create high quality, safe and innovative maternity services to women in this province has dissolved into a colossal waste of time, energy and money on the part of all concerned, including the Quebec taxpayers" (Stonier and Beauchemin 1993).

The dominant status of the medical and nursing professions is not likely to be set aside in maternity and infant care. Virtually all nation-states actively promote medical and nursing education and practice, and there is a strong case for further developing the knowledge base and clinical practices associated with the medical and nursing professions. A related point concerns the artificiality of some constraints on birth attendants. As was set out in chapter three, the monopoly powers of the various provincial medical associations and their colleges have been achieved, in part, through the denunication and prosecution of the predecessors of today's midwives. The issues ahead will revolve around whether current midwifery initiatives are co-opted by the established health professions in Canada and who controls licensure, training, and peer review.

NURSING AND MIDWIFERY:
"EVERYTHING THAT RISES
MUST CONVERGE"

For the most part, midwifery has been seen as having a different role from that of nursing. As a calling or as a profession, midwifery usually stands alone and apart from nursing education and employment worldwide. There are signs, however, of a convergence and alliance-making between nursing associations and midwifery associations. In the United States nurse-midwifery was established as a combination of the two spheres. Chapter 1 described several differences between accredited nurse-midwives and community midwives in North America. As a rule, nurse-midwives work as salaried employees in hospital or clinic settings. They belong to professional nursing associations. Nurse-midwives are usually not responsible for intensive in-home prenatal care of clients, nor do they usually assume responsibility for the delivery stage of childbirth. Nurse-midwifery in Canada is usually associated with pilot projects such as the Low-Risk Clinic in Vancouver. In the United States, however, nurse-midwifery is more established.

Stereotyping nurse-midwives as a group is hazardous. There is great variation in the sphere of practice, especially in northern regions where midwives may be responsible for many decisions ordinarily assumed by medical personnel. In this chapter, the role of nurse-midwives is evaluated, with special attention to community midwifery practice. Significant initiatives are discussed: the attempt to establish an out-of-hospital birthing clinic in Vancouver, the Low-Risk Clinic, which allowed more independent practice and continuity of care by nurse-midwives, and the succeeding Midwives' Project at the Grace Hospital in Vancouver.

Central Problems in Nurse-Midwifery

Whatever the attempts to promote midwifery services, it is not uncommon for nurse-midwives to express resentment at the containment of their skills in attending women in childbirth. For some, the opportunity to apply these skills is truncated when they arrive in urban settings where physicians are dominant within the occupational hierarchy of hospitals. A midwife (and nurse) working in Canada but trained in England, remarked on the structure of obstetrical care and the limits placed on trained midwives: "I worked on the obstetrical unit (of a 55-bed hospital in the North). That was really interesting; I did quite a few deliveries because the medical coverage wasn't always that great. And basically I worked autonomously, with some limitations ... I was allowed a lot of freedom to practise in my own way. I think if I had not had that I would have found it very limiting. The physicians who were there were very inexperienced in obstetrics ... I realized why I was necessary, why they made a prerequisite of midwifery training for anyone who worked on the obstetrical unit ... they really needed my skills ... The most shocking experience I ever had in Canada was when I worked in a university hospital. Every woman had an obstetrician. It was a high-risk unit, but many of these women were not high risk. There were 18 obstetricians on staff. Women literally came in and had birth done to them."

The leitmotif of professionalism that appears throughout the definitions of nurse-midwifery has been criticized. A few community midwives have expressed their misgivings about what they see as the proprietary nature of some obstetrical nurses, managing the baby as their "property" while disciplining errant parents and community midwives. By contrast, some practitioners praise nurse-midwives for taking time with patients, for combining this rapport with clinical skills that are at least on a par with medical staff. Midwives' enthusiasm for continuity of care for expectant women may also clash with a medical model of birth in which labour and delivery may be disparaged as time-consuming, unexciting "handholding" (Scully 1980, 125–6). The movement for greater recognition of nurse-midwives as birth attendants has contributed to an expanded role in conventional obstetrical settings. The recent proliferation of nurse-midwifery programs in the United States (Scupholme 1982, 21). has often been interpreted in terms of consumer demand for alternatives to standard obstetrical attendance at birth. Midwives are active in tertiary care, and can collaborate with obstetricans and anaestheologists over decisions about pain relief in obstetrical care (Ghosh-Ray et al. 1980). A

survey of practising midwives in the United States in 1976, which
gathered data on 1,213 nurse-midwives, confirmed that the collaboration between physicians and nurse-midwives permitted a degree
of treatment of birth complications by nurse-midwives. This survey
found that only 15 per cent of nurse-midwives working in the general
area of deliveries managed multiple births. Only 12 per cent were
responsible for breech deliveries. Nevertheless, 99 per cent of certified
nurse-midwives (CNMs) performed and repaired episiotomies: "In
general, the more invasive and risky the procedure, the less likely
nurse-midwives are to perform it. However, nearly as many (89 per
cent) reported they managed the care of prenatal patients with some
complications. A number of minor complications occur quite commonly in otherwise normal pregnancies, creating a gray area between
'normal, well, uncomplicated patients' and 'high-risk' or 'complicated' patients. Most nurse-midwives providing prenatal care have
developed collaborative relationships with physicians in which they
can continue to care for patients who experience certain kinds of
prenatal complications" (Rooks and Fischman 1980, 992–3).

One difference frequently suggested in the literature is that independent (community) midwives are more politicized than nurse-
midwives. There appears to be a subcultural approach by some
community midwives, including a resolve to respect the woman's
wishes during labour and delivery and throughout the pregnancy
and post-partum period. The community midwife, according to this
portrait, is more likely to regard organized medicine as profit-
oriented and male-dominated. In her practice she may contravene
local or international practice guidelines on the basis of her judgment
of the situation and out of respect for the women. This appears to
be linked with two major themes: the historical takeover of birth by
physicians from community midwives, and the perception that
nurse-midwives are greatly constrained within the hospital hierarchy
and unable to apply their skills fully to the women they serve. Cobb
(1981, 75) indicates that nurse-midwives have been coopted by the
dominant medical profession. One British Columbia community midwife observed that nurse-midwifery is less threatening to physicians'
power than autonomous midwifery: "One reason why physicians
want it to be nurse-midwifery is that they know how to control
nurses, and they train nurses to be under their control. Physicians
are terrified of the independent midwife who does a three-year program, and isn't a nurse. They are afraid of that woman because she
doesn't do what they say ... If they have to have midwives, and it
looks like they will, then they want to have nurse-midwives. They
don't want to lose their piece of the pie to midwives. The only way

they can prevent that is to insist that every midwife have a physician present when she does a delivery."

The subcultural motif may be overdrawn with respect to many community midwives as well as nurse-midwives. My impression is that midwives tend to be oriented toward a community of clients and not toward a particular community or locality. In fact, the great majority of home births analysed in this study took place in over two hundred localities throughout Ontario, British Columbia, and Saskatchewan. It is also unsupportable to juxtapose community midwives against nurse-midwives as if the latter were not also serving a community or constituency. That constituency would tend to be disinclined to home birth and to be fairly positive toward conventional management of childbirth by physicians and nurses. There are instances of nurses taking action outside the conventional hospital network. There are of course exceptions; for example, an Ontario nurse published a favourable account of her decision to give birth at home with medical attendance (see Swedlo 1979, 307–53). Starr (1983, 223) holds that even in the seventeenth and eighteenth centuries in the United States, the lay midwife was regarded as a competitor by many medical men, while the nurse-midwife was not. Others are in agreement that nurse-midwifery in the United States is primarily a dependent occupation: "It is perhaps a mistake to refer to midwifery in the United States as an emerging profession. Midwifery as it was known in Europe and England never really existed; decisions, political and economic, were made which led to the elimination of midwifery. What is slowly emerging is a health worker called a nurse-midwife – an asssistant to the obstetrician and not an independent practitioner. Only 10 per cent of American nurse-midwives are presently employed in positions that offer full use of their training" (Anisef and Basson 1979, 368).

Another difference between modern community midwifery and nurse-midwifery involves the apprenticeship in birth attendance. Unlike the formal training in midwifery, usually in conjunction with completion of nursing training, community midwives tend to learn by practical experience unsupported by formal training: that is, through attending births and reading birth manuals. This differentiation between midwives trained in nursing and other midwives can in turn be linked to comments on the "proletarianization" of nursing (Wagner 1980) and the deflection of u.s. nurses' efforts to achieve greater autonomy. A related point is that solidarity among nurses in Canada is narrowly defined (Buckley 1979). Deference to medical authority is pronounced, although the emergence of provincial and national organizations and of collective bargaining status has countered this historical situation. In Canada, the direction of legal lobbying and professional recognition has been toward an expanded role of certified nurse-midwives. It is estimated that there are at least one hundred certified nurse-midwives in British Columbia (Brook 1980, 6). Independent midwifery practice has generally been restricted to nurses working in remote regions with limited or non-existent access to physicians. A midwifery program at the master's level has been offered at Memorial University. An advanced obstetrical nursing course is continuing at the University of Alberta, and outpost nursing, with a midwifery component, is available at Dalhousie University in Halifax, Nova Scotia.

The movement toward a more independent practice for midwives in Canada was favoured by Louise Miner, past president of the Canadian Nurses' Association. She criticized general practitioners for simultaneously acknowledging their limitations while resisting midwifery practice. Normal pregnancies should be attended by midwives, and midwives should practice independently (see Korcok 1972, 45). In 1971 a survey of members of the Society of Obstetricians and Gynecologists of Canada found that the majority of members responding to the survey accepted the premise of trained midwives taking more responsibility in prenatal and antenatal care. Nevertheless, there was a general reluctance to give midwives the primary responsibility for managing the delivery of babies. Concern was also expressed about a possible lack of supervision by physicians of midwives in maternity practice (Korcok 1972a, 7). This reluctance to endorse nurse-midwives as birth attendants is also evident in the drafting of a document concerning the regionalization of maternity and newborn care in the United States. The American College of Nurse-Midwives (ACNM) was not invited to contribute to the drafting of this document (see Sugarman 1979, 69).

A statement in support of nurse-midwifery practice was adopted by the Registered Nurses Association of British Columbia in June 1979, following a ten-month investigation by a three-member committee. This statement included resolutions that the role of the nurse-practitioner should be established in British Columbia; that the practice of nurse-midwifery should be legally defined as "part of the ordinary calling of nursing," thereby securing an exemption from prosecution under section 71 of the Medical Practitioners Act; that standards of nurse-midwifery practice should be met; that various types of practice could be subsumed, including domiciliary (home) births and management of low-risk and high-risk births in hospitals or clinics; and that refresher courses be made available for nurse-midwives (RNABC, 1979). In 1993, certain representations made to the Health Professions Council of British Columbia were hostile to the concept of home births and to the autonomy of midwives (that is, to their working without the direct supervision of physicians). The midwives' representatives countered that such supervision constituted a costly and unnecessary duplication of services.

Home Birth and Midwifery Policy

The issue of home birth has generated some consensus on the preferability of hospital settings for delivery. The Western Nurse-Midwives Association registered its preference for working with obstetricians in clinical settings (Canadian Press 1976). A spokeswoman for the Registered Nurses' Association of British Columbia stated the association's opposition to home deliveries as an alternative to hospital deliveries, adding that inadequate back-up services in British Columbia did not allow for safe home deliveries. The spokeswoman added that this policy position does not discredit home birth per se but instead emphasizes the importance of not undertaking domiciliary obstetrics without established access to emergency back-up services. The concept of nurse-midwives working in hospital settings, supervised by physicians, was recently endorsed by a joint committee of representatives from the Registered Nurses' Association of British Columbia and from the College of Physicians and Surgeons (Padmore 1983, A7).

Another potential area of conflict between midwives involves attempts to legitimize community midwifery practice. The Midwives Alliance of North America (MANA) comprises nurse-midwives and community midwives, and the Midwives' Association of British Columbia encourages membership of nurse-midwives and community midwives. Nevertheless, some certified nurse-midwife members have opposed the lack of clear standards of education and practice for community midwives (Campbell 1982). MANA representatives have sought to establish standards for "basic competency" for certified nurse-midwives and community midwives alike (Ventre and Leonard 1982, 23–4). The tension between certified midwives and other midwives is linked with a general trend toward professionalized health care, including nursing. Midwives may be concerned that the institutional structures of hospital-based births (with physicians and managers directing and assessing midwives' work) may undermine midwifery services (Kitzinger 1988, 10). There seems to be a tendency for certain tasks to be delegated to subordinates as organizations become more complex: for example, record-keeping and scheduling, once deemed the bailiwick of doctors, have been delegated to nursing staff (see Hughes et al. 1958, 7; Growe 1991, 103).

Alternative Birth Centres

The introduction of alternative birth centres (ABCS) as a compromise between domiciliary birth settings and obstetrical wards is one example of innovation that results, in part, from consumer demands for the humanistic and flexible management of pregnancy and childbirth. For example, staff at a free-standing birth centre in Culver City, California, encourage families to remain together throughout labour. Women often choose a variety of delivery positions in these centres. Certified nurse-midwives are employed in the centre (Mittelbach 1986, 10). This apparently neat equation of birth innovations and public demands does not take into account the historic rivalry between various professional and non-professional associations (Freidson 1972). Nor does it address suggestions that ABCS do not significantly alter the incidence of obstetrical interventions.

With direct reference to alternative birth centres, DeVries (1980) contends that the apparent freedom accorded patients in ABCS is in fact used to consolidate the power of birth centre staff. Notwithstanding the homelike decor and espousal of unmedicated births, where possible, ABCS are characterized by unjustifiably high rates of invasive treatment, including analgesia, anaesthesia, episiotomy, and forceps delivery. DeVries (1984, 98) cites one study that documented a transfer rate of 46 per cent of patients from an alternative birth centre to a conventional labour and delivery suite. A televised documentary on home birth in the United States indicated that between 20 and 50 per cent of women entering an ABC will be transferred to operating rooms for forceps delivery, caesarean section, electronic fetal monitoring, and so forth (CBS News 1982). Establishment of birthing rooms within hospitals is another method of adapting settings to consumer demands, although it has been reported that in some hospitals the birthing rooms account for only a small proportion (in some cases as low as 3 per cent) of all births in hospital.

Some disagree that ABCS are in the best interest of pregnant women and infants. The growth of birth centres is tied to the professional interest of nurse-midwives, long subordinated to doctors' control through denial of hospital privileges and inadequate back-up services. The negative assessment of alternative birth centres (ABCS) is far from universal. Rothman (1983, 3–7) acknowledges that women giving birth in ABCS report satisfaction with their care.

Another point of concern arises from the failure to establish out-of-hospital birthing centres. An earlier proposal to develop an out-of-hospital clinic in Vancouver was not accepted by a federal funding agency. It was suggested by one person involved in the proposal that the lack of support among physicians was a factor in rejecting the clinic proposal.

Conclusion

Historically, midwifery programs in Newfoundland, Nova Scotia, Quebec, and Alberta "were designed to prepare nurses and others to care for mothers and babies in isolated areas" (Herbert 1993, 4; see also Field 1991, 5). With the decision to legalize midwifery in some Canadian provinces, midwifery training will provide a broader base of practice, such that qualified midwives will practise in urban as well as rural and northern settings. Broader access to midwifery training is also important. In Ontario the Bachelor of Health Science (Midwifery) program offered at McMaster University, Ryerson Polytechnical Institute, and Laurentian University provides for distance-education courses (in English or French at Laurentian). The program "will hold a number of spaces for aboriginal students" (Herbert 1993, 4). Such provisions are meant to increase access to training for prospective midwives. Relyea (1992, 168) favours midwifery programs that foster "the admittance of persons from a variety of backgrounds and educational preparation." In future, midwives will probably resemble Lesley Page's (1993, 1483–5) vision of the expert and "experienced clinician" who is aware of the available scientific literature and is able to act as a companion for expectant mothers.

MIDWIFERY DEMONSTRATION PROJECTS

The Low-Risk Clinic (originally called the "Hands-On Clinic for Nurse Instructors") was a pilot project that operated at the Grace Hospital in Vancouver from September 1981 until May 1984. The program remains in place in the new Grace Hospital in Vancouver, with six midwifery staff at the core of the project. It is now called the Midwifery Program. It is useful to look at the findings from one report published in the 1980s by those involved with this initiative.

In the Low-Risk Clinic, four nurse-midwives and four obstetricians worked together in caring for sixty-one women. This pilot project in a major hospital in Canada's third largest city was designed to provide safe deliveries of babies, to demonstrate the competency of

Table 18
Mode of Delivery

Mode of delivery	Low-Risk Clinic		Grace Hospital	
	N	%	N	%
Spontaneous	40	73.0	na	58.7
Forceps	9	16.0	na	19.8
Caesarean	6	11.0	na	21.5
Total	55	100.0	na	100.0

Source: Elaine Carty et al., *The Low-Risk Clinic* (1984: 25).

trained nurse-midwives in managing births with fewer interventions than occurred in conventional birth attendance. Continuity of care was sought. Extensive prenatal care was provided by the midwives, along with consultation with the physicians and nursing staff. It is important to note that the four women acting as midwives volunteered their time. In contrast, the current Midwifery Program involves one full-time staff member; another full-time position is split between two (part-time) staff. In addition, there is a director subsumed within the division of nursing at Grace Hospital.

The report on this project generally confirms the viability of more independent midwifery practice within a major hospital. A follow-up survey indicated that the clients were generally pleased with the project. One measure of the success of the project was the increased rate of spontaneous vaginal deliveries among the Low-Risk Clinic patients in comparison with hospital-wide statistics (see table 18). (As noted earlier, approximately 93 per cent of the attempted home births attended by the community midwives resulted in spontaneous vaginal deliveries.)

The report provides a useful description of specific policies and procedures for assessing the health of the woman and fetus throughout the pregnancy, as well as procedures for consultation with pediatricians, general practititoners, obstretricians, and nursing staff. An integral purpose of the clinic was to accommodate the wishes of the couple where possible and to ensure safe deliveries. The success of the Low-Risk Clinic led to the development of the subsequent Midwifery Project in the Grace Hospital. This ongoing project is an established part of the labour and delivery budget at the hospital. A midwife working in this service believed that such projects can be supported by physicians, and can benefit the obstetrical staff generally: "Exemplary nurse-physician relationships are alive in Vancouver. Our experience with one general practitioner in the midwifery service at Grace Hospital is the best. Not only does this particular physician donate time and energy to the program, he supports and stands up for the midwifery cause, controversial as it is" (Robertson 1990, 5).

A pilot study of labour coaching by midwives in Toronto General Hospital supported the premise that midwife-assisted births provided fewer interventions than physician-managed births. The use of epidurals, forceps, and episiotomies was lower in the midwife-assisted sample (n = 51) than in the physician-managed sample (n = 58), although only the episiotomy rates (38 per cent and 18 per cent, respectively) achieved statistical significance. The pilot study supports findings from other studies in which intervention rates were found to be lowered through the involvement of midwives (Reid and Galbraith 1988, 1989–90). Although there is no systematic update of community midwives' work in British Columbia, the results described in this chapter correspond closely with birth statistics compiled by Carol-Anne Letty, a licensed midwife who has a home birth practice in Vancouver. Reviewing outcomes for home births (n = 30) and hospital births (n = 8) between July 1991 and June 1993, she noted that none of the thirty women who gave birth at home had had episiotomies. There were three caesarean sections, and the remainder delivered on their hands and knees (n = 18), semi-sitting (n = 10), side-lying (n = 4), and with a birthing stool (n = 3). No infant deaths occurred in this sample (Letty 1993).

A continuing difficulty in assessing the nature of contemporary birth attendance, including attendance in alternative birth centres, is the lack of information on particular centres. To some extent this lack has been overcome by recently published accounts of birth centres and nurse-midwifery practice in hospital settings in the United States. Several of these published accounts will be outlined here to indicate general themes and to underscore difficulties associated with evaluation studies from California, Arizona, Georgia, and Florida. These selected studies provide additional evidence in support of the safety of nurse-midwifery practice. More recent research has been interpreted very favourably with respect to birthing centres (see Lubic 1992). Perinatal mortality rates are lower than the average rate in the respective states and well within expected rates of perinatal mortality generally. There also tends to be a reduction in caesarean section rates, forceps deliveries, and the use of anaesthesia.

The incommensurability of these reports highlights a general difficulty of reportage (see also Wagner 1985, 114–15). Although reportage usually centres on conventional variables such as birth outcome, obstetrical interventions, and infant mortality and morbidity, there is nevertheless a tendency toward unstandardized reportage wherein certain variables are presented and others omitted, without a clear statement of why some are deemed salient to the comparison of (nurse) midwifery practice with other birth attendants. This unstandardized method of reportage, along with missing data, impedes comparisons of findings pertaining to nurse-midwifery services.

The demonstration projects address a central tenet in the continuing debate over midwifery attendance: that midwifery attendance is uniquely suited to uncomplicated births. It has been asserted that "nurse-midwives are cost-effective because we can show improved neonatal and maternal outcomes with fewer medical interventions, because we provide safe births in less expensive out-of-hospital settings or for fewer hospital days, and because we can show that emotional support and education about nutrition, exercise, breast-feeding, and self-care are worthwhile" (Kraus 1984, 2). Haire (1981) contends that nurse-midwifery practice is superior to conventional medical attendance in many respects, particularly in promoting unmedicated births and reducing the incidence of episiotomies and instrumental deliveries. Haire combines her observations of maternity hospitals in Great Britain, Russia, western Europe, and elsewhere with more detailed observations of nurse-midwifery practice in the North Central Bronx Hospital, the Frontier Nursing Service in Kentucky, and the Su Clinica Familia in Texas. With specific reference to the North Central Bronx Hospital, of 2,608 midwife-assisted births in 1979, a relatively high percentage (88 per cent) delivered vaginally and spontaneously. Analgesia or anesthesia was resorted to in less than 30 per cent of all labours, while forceps and vacuum extraction together accounted for just over 2 per cent of deliveries. Over a third of women attempting a vaginal birth after a caesarean (VBAC) did so successfully. Nearly half (45 per cent) of births were done over an intact perineum, 26 per cent required episiotomies, and 29 per cent involved lacerations (a fourth-degree laceration occurred in 1 per cent of births studied). Haire's (1981) estimation of the importance of contemporary nurse-midwifery attendance is further reinforced by a study of a nurse-midwifery program in a county hospital in rural California. That study documented significant decreases in the rate of prematurity (from 11 per cent to 6.6 per cent) and the rate of neonatal mortality (from 23.9 per cent to 10.3 per cent) during the period (1961 to 1963) in which the nurse-midwives were active. Two additional points are of interest: first, such dramatic changes in these rates were not manifested in other regions of the county during the operation of the nurse-midwifery program; second, rates of prematurity and neonatal mortality increased significantly after the program was discontinued. Among other factors, the researchers suggest that women receiving care during the three-year program were more likely to receive prenatal care and to begin prenatal contact earlier (Levy et al. 1971). This special status accorded nurse-midwives appears also in a recent discussion on malpractice liability of nurse-midwives. Certified nurse-midwives differ in terms of client satisfaction and participation, while the CNM's expertise and reputation for safety is retained. Nevertheless, litigation against American nurse-midwives increased in the 1980s, and is expected to continue as midwives widen their ambit of practice (Sinquefield 1983).

Nurse-midwifery practice in Canada, the United States, Britain, and elsewhere is characterized by the movement toward professionalized health care. The professional standard of care is achieved through specialized instruction (academic and practical), supervision by governing bodies such as nursing colleges and specialized associations, and the formulation of overarching standards of patient care. Just as midwives face contradictions in health structures (see Kitzinger 1988), so also are nurses subject to pressures of overwork and counter-pressures to recognize the value of their work and their ability to function more autonomously (Growe 1991). There are also pressures to develop feminist-based curricula in nursing, and to highlight the exclusion of some visible minorities from the profession (see Hedin and Donovan 1989; hooks 1989).

The current status of midwives with nursing accreditation may well be rising above the sometimes disparaged status of obstetrical nursing (see Hughes et al. 1958, 85). Nevertheless, in terms of prestige it is still conventionally ranked well below the medical specialties such as obstetrics (Lin 1976).

MIDWIFERY PRACTICE AND FORMAL AUTHORITY

The contradiction between professional training and the formally subordinate status of nurse-midwifery (whereby nurse-midwives may be supervised by doctors in order to practise) may lead to informal, covert tactics to circumvent legal and professional strictures on practice (see Hughes et al. 1958, 64–72, 172–3). These informal tactics may be quite effective in allowing midwives to practise their skills and in reducing interventions deemed unnecessary by the midwives. An important point, however, is that the circumvention of physicians' authority is substantively different from direct challenges to a physician's judgment. Concerns about professional prestige can be linked with the manner in which formal authority impinges on, or threatens to impinge on, midwifery practice. Midwifery practice is subject to a variety of cultural, legal, and social rules in British Columbia and other provinces. It is important to remember, however, that midwives can circumvent some of the intrusions of technology and official gatekeeping. Direct challenges to official authority are sometimes avoided through appeals to orthodox authority, even fictional ones. A senior community midwife offered this vignette: "I did a birth up in Lund, near Powell River. I flew up there. The only problem I had, and this was something I hadn't considered, was that I had to fly from Vancouver International Airport and I had to go through the metal detector machine. And so the security officer said 'What's this?' when the birth kit was detected. I was quite embarrassed and I wasn't quite sure how to explain myself. I wound up saying that my husband was a doctor and that I was taking some equipment up there for him."

Passing through an airport checkpoint is one obstacle; the threat of prosecution for criminal or quasi-criminal offences is quite another. The following excerpt from an interview with a senior community midwife illustrates some dynamics of state measures of power and offsetting resources drawn upon by a midwife under official scrutiny.

The only time the legality issue came up for me was with a birth several years after I began doing primary care births. I had a really bad feeling about this birth and for the first time of all the births I attended I had three other primary care midwives assisting me with this birth. I still had this bad feeling but I couldn't pinpoint anything to screen her out (from attempting a home birth). Even her physician said I was being paranoid.

Anyway, the birth was fine and the baby was fine. Afterward I wondered why I had been so uptight about this birth. On the fifth day the mother called me to say that her baby had died in her sleep. I should have said that she shouldn't call anyone, the police, ambulance – until I arrived.

It was a 20-minute drive to her place and when I arrived the police and ambulance were already there. Now, the unfortunate thing is that my client was a single mother on welfare and the police officers treated her badly, suspiciously. It was completely out of the question that this woman would have injured her daughter. The police officers found out that the baby had been delivered at home, with a midwife present, and by the time I walked in the door they had been given my name. I took the mother to the morgue to see the child. When we returned the police wanted to question us in separate rooms.

I was asked a few questions off the record. The policeman didn't understand this situation. He said, "Who's illegal here? Is she (the mother) illegal?

Are you illegal?" "Who's in trouble?" is essentially what he was asking. I explained that midwifery is illegal and that if anyone was in trouble it would be me for practising midwifery without a licence. The police officer then asked me if I was a midwife. I said, "Do you think I should answer that, or do you think it would be really incriminating?" He said that I probably shouldn't answer, and he agreed with me that the mother probably shouldn't answer any more questions at this time.

The mother needed to talk. She wanted to settle these questions immediately. But when the officers said they wanted to take her to the station for questioning, I said "forget it." The mother was grieving, she was very shocky. The officers were angry with me for protecting her and said that they would get to me next, and that I would have to go to the police station. They asked the mom if she had beaten her baby – there were no marks on her body and I knew they didn't have any right to take her anywhere. I told them to get out. The mother wanted to be interviewed, however, in the house, so I told her not to answer any more questions. I glanced down at the officer's sheet. There were two questions: Was she your midwife? (she said yes) and did you pay her? (yes). The last question made me feel "Oh man, I'm in trouble."

That night I cleared out birth records, equipment, books from my house. It is frightening to think of having my records confiscated by the police: the records are invaluable to a midwife. I was informed by the police that I would be charged with criminal negligence causing death. They were awaiting the results of the autopsy report. It took 48 hours for the report to be completed and the conclusion was that the baby died of SIDS [sudden infant death syndrome]. Then I was threatened with a possible charge of practising medicine without a licence under the Medical Practitioners Act.

I was so relieved that the criminal charge had been dropped. The Midwives' Association of B.C. held an emergency meeting to discuss strategies if I was charged under the Medical Practitioners Act. I was enthusiastic about the trial. We decided that we would encourage consumer picketing of the trial, and that we should invite experts from Holland and the U.S.A. to speak to the issue of medical monopolization of birth in this province. However, my client contacted me after a visit from the police. She was told that the charge against me would be dropped. Now, they had plenty of evidence against me: her statement, for instance, and I had provided documentation of the birth (Apgar scores, and other details). My understanding was that the British Columbia Medical Association representatives were unwilling to launch a prosecution that would rally support for midwifery. I think that they wanted to make me sweat about it, but the charge never materialized.

This account draws together a few central themes in the control of deviance and legal measures. The first is that there are points of support that the midwife could call upon: careful documentation of prenatal care, labour, delivery, and prenatal visits; her efforts to check on the mother's and infant's health (through the physician and the presence of three other midwives); and her cooperation with the authorities up to a point. It also dramatizes her suspicion of police activities. At another point in the interview she confided that she had destroyed numerous birth records after a (false) rumour that her house might be searched for evidence. In retrospect, she said she might have stored them safely away, but this would raise new problems, including confidentiality.

The broader point of support is the resources of the Midwives' Association, and, beyond that, plans to involve other practitioners in a direct challenge to the illegal status of midwifery in British Columbia. It seems that this is a clear example of of the danger of assuming that midwives are defenceless against official powers of the state and the interests of the medical profession. Women do organize against some restrictions on reproductive rights, as evidenced a variety of associations that represent or support midwives. These include the Association of Ontario Midwives, the Midwives Association of British Columbia, the Alberta Association of Midwives, the Midwives Association of Saskatchewan, the Association of Nova Scotia Midwives, the Midwifery Coalition of Nova Scotia, the Association des Sages Femmes du Québec, the Alliance Québécoise des Sages-Femmes Practiciennes, Naissance-Renaissance, the Alliance of Nurse-Midwives, the Maternity and Neonatal Nurses of Newfoundland and Labrador, the Midwives Association of North America (MANA), the Canadian Confederation of Midwives, and so forth (Canadian Confederation of Midwives 1992).

The general principle that the state ought not interfere in private matters without good reason is also a check on state intrusion, especially in the ordinarily private sphere of reproduction and family relationships (Burtch et al. 1985). Parents may act as a resource for midwives by vouching for the midwife, protecting her, and threatening to embarrass officials. The following is extracted from an interview with a community midwife in the mid-1980s.

Q: Have you ever had pressure or interest expressed in your work by the police or the courts?

A: Every time the medical profession [in a city outside the Lower Mainland area] caught wind of my attending a home birth they reported it to the British Columbia Medical Association, the RCMP [Royal Canadian Mounted Police], or both. I had a situation with a very fast, a precipitate birth with a woman who was a VBAC [vaginal birth after caesarean section]. The couple was over an hour from a major hospital and while I didn't agree outright to assist at a home birth, I said that I would respect the woman's wishes. I left their house while the woman was in labour, just to visit my children who were nearby, and I was called back because the woman was pushing.

By the time the other midwife and I returned, it was a precipitate birth, a good portion of the baby's head was showing. At birth, the baby was totally "shocky" [in shock]. We resuscitated the baby – which wasn't difficult to do in this case – and as a standard procedure in CPR we called for an ambulance. The paramedics took 20 minutes to get there and they were no help. I asked them to wait until the placenta had been delivered. (This was a precipitate delivery and there is a greater chance of hemorrhage with these deliveries). They asked "was this a planned birth?" and just snooped around the house. Then they said they couldn't stay in the house because they both had to listen to the radio (dispatches) in the ambulance.

What happened after that was that doctors, on reviewing the ambulance calls for that month, reported this incident to the police and the BCMA [British Columbia Medical Association]. The police visited the mother several times. Every time the mother referred to me as "her friend." [She would say] "It was lucky that my friend was there." She also promised to pull apart the ambulance service publicly. I got a real sense of persecution ... To be on the safe side I moved my supplies and birth records to a friend's house. This was the only real occasion that the police were involved: I am aware that the BCMA and the police were contacted on a couple of other occasions, but nothing happened.

This account underlines the ways in which prosecutorial power can be restricted. An autopsy report that would be ammunition for the defence is pertinent here, just as the lack of witnesses and other events can hinder prosecution efforts (Osborne 1983). On a far broader level, midwives have received out-and-out support from such groups as the International Childbirth Education Association and the Federation of University Women (Ontario 1992).

It is a mistake, however, to exaggerate the powers of community midwives. Action has been taken against practising midwives in British Columbia, Ontario, and Nova Scotia; charges were contemplated, then dropped, against midwives involved in the delivery of twins in Winnipeg in 1990. Community midwifery is primarily affiliated with home birth (although some community midwives also provide labour coaching in hospital and prenatal classes), and their clientele is quite limited in number. Only about 1 per cent of births in contemporary British Columbia occur out of hospital, and a number of these are not planned home births. There is thus a considerable difference between the situation of the community midwife in British Columbia and that of the village midwives in Third World countries, where a great proportion of birthing in outlying areas is managed by traditional midwives (see Peng et al. 1972, 25–8).

The dominant cultural perspective on childbirth emphasizes risk to the mother and infant, the superiority of professional medical and nursing attendance, and the value of institutionalized birthing in hospital settings. Community midwives have drawn on a variety of evaluation studies of the place of birth and the issue of safety to argue against the assumption of greater safety in hospitals; they have also relied on their own experience in assisting thousands of Canadian women to give birth over the past two decades. This said, the cultural emphasis on hospital deliveries remains deeply rooted today and is unlikely to be substantially dislodged in the future.

The practice of midwifery is connected with legal rules surrounding childbirth, which are in turn closely aligned with the state authority. In a politically organized society, laws are ostensibly made in the public interest. This is quite clear with respect to the formulation of provincial medical acts in Canada. Such legislation affords medical practitioners a monopoly status over a variety of diagnostic and clinical activities; it also vests in physicians considerable powers of professional self-regulation through disciplinary hearings concerning professional misconduct and alleged incompetence. Time and again such monopolistic legislation is defended on the basis that it serves to protect the public interest. Professional monopoly status should ensure the highest level of training and peer scrutiny. Clearly, this presumption cuts across another cultural belief in the value of competition as it may affect standards, along with the freedom to choose one's occupation. It is evident that as work has become more professionalized and bureaucratized, the legal regulation of work has heightened. This regulation includes the attempt by occupational groupings to secure their market status by excluding rival groupings (Reasons and Chappell 1985; Giddens 1982, 188). Alternative groupings such as the Midwives' Association of British Columbia are more likely to be assessed in terms of their "integrative function" – that is, the intrinsic value of such groups as perceived by their members. These alternative groups nevertheless must contend with extrinsic factors that encouraged their members to become more professional, to establish standards, to be governed by other more established organizations such as a nurses' college (Light 1981).

There is an overt political dimension to some varieties of lay midwifery. A common theme is that obstetrical knowledge is deliberately restricted to medical (and nursing) personnel, that alternative practitioners continue to be outlawed while a medical monopoly is preserved, and that profit and male dominance in the structure of health care are an integral part of current childbirth practices. This critique is accompanied by the advocacy of collective, non-hierarchical options for women seeking to practice health care and for their clients. It may also be extended to caution midwives about accepting the dominant methods of evaluating midwifery care. The danger, it is said, is that women giving birth, and their attendants, can have their experiences distorted by "scientific" studies of birth management (see generally Kirby and McKenna 1989).

SUMMARY

Studies of community midwifery practice and of the practices of "legal" midwives active in birthing centres and hospitals in the United States lend weight to the argument that midwifery care can be beneficial for women giving birth and their infants. In Canada, community midwives appear to be successful in reducing rates of instrumental delivery; similarly, they appear to achieve results comparable or superior to those of conventional hospital-based deliveries in terms of infant mortality and morbidity. Nonetheless, there are some deficiencies in the informal practice of midwifery, and instances of unsafe home birth practices have been reported.

For nurse-midwives, there is little to support past or present allegations that their work is inferior to physician-presided birth attendance. Indeed, there is decisive evidence that nurse-midwives can contribute in tertiary care as well as primary care settings. With respect to the community midwifery movement, however, there is concern that unregulated midwives may practise outside safety guidelines. Some infant deaths in Canada have been attributed, at least in part, to unsatisfactory midwifery. Community midwives operate without the protection of a Midwives Act and without the material resources and organizational structures available to their medical and nursing counterparts. Moreover, when they initiate midwifery practices or establish a midwifery school they face the threat of prosecution or the problem of limited funding.

The significance of the community midwifery movement can be linked with other attempts to decentralize institutionalized processes, including the management of death in hospices or at home, the victims' rights movement in criminal justice, and efforts to establish alternative (informal) dispute resolution through mediation (Christie 1978). The situation of nurse-midwives in many jurisdictions is complex, inasmuch as they are often highly trained and often assist fully in uncomplicated deliveries. In Canada, however, their presence has been and continues to be fairly restricted. The current attempts to establish demonstration projects have been only partly successful. The proposal to staff a clinic outside a hospital setting was not accepted in 1979, and the Low-Risk Clinic in the Grace Hospital has been replaced by a different structure in which nurse-midwives do not provide the same continuity of care to expectant mothers. The clinic is nonetheless a recognition that the nurse-midwife's conventional role can be expanded in response to consumer demand and to lobbying for greater autonomy from within the nursing profession. Muzio (1991) favours a cooperative model whereby midwives define their own educational programs and work collaboratively with nurses.

While resistance to the hegemonic powers of the state and the professions is evident, the end result is not a marked diminution of those powers. The following chapter reconsiders legal regulation of midwifery practice in Canada; chapter 6 examines the future of world midwifery services.

CHAPTER FIVE

Midwives and the Law

INTRODUCTION

A trial of labour, in obstetrical terminology, refers to a situation where a woman may not be able to deliver vaginally because of suspected cephalopelvic disproportion, or where a woman has previously given birth by caesarean section and is being "allowed" to labour for a prescribed period of time before intervention (Cohen 1991). This terminology seems apropos for midwives in conflict with the law in Canada. Unproved, not yet established, and open to suspicion for their practices and motives, midwives in Canadian jurisdictions face an unsettled, tentative situation in law and in the health-care system. The medical profession and state authorities have become gatekeepers in the supervision and vetting of women's choices in reproduction.

This chapter provides a detailed look at key cases that have shaped the midwifery movement. While the focus is on Canadian cases heard in the past decade, it is important to consider the earlier discussion of how laws and medical ideology coincided so as to eliminate or vastly restrict midwifery practice in Canada and many other countries. According to the midwives themselves, what they are seeking is not an opportunity to prove themselves within the limits of pilot projects or short-term experiments, but recognition of their skills. By and large, their efforts have been bent toward respecting women's wishes – whether the women wish to give birth in a private setting or with a crowd, and whether they wish to give birth at home, in hospital, or in intermediate settings such as alternative birth centres.

A common denominator for midwives actively involved in the Midwifery Task Force of British Columbia and the Midwives Association of British Columbia is the desire for legalized, autonomous midwifery. Few midwives are willing to continue to practise without an assurance that the law will not be invoked against them. The threat of criminal prosecution, a coroner's investigation, or charges of practising medicine without a licence is ever-present for community midwives. This discouraging of midwives and their supporters is not peculiar to Canada. Odent (1986, 133) notes that in the western world doctors supportive of home birth often face professional criticism. He adds: "With the training of midwives as it is at the moment, not only are we not getting authentic midwives, but we are often stopping the careers at an early stage of those women who genuinely want to help other women at birth. This is done either by hassles with authority, or because it is hard to earn your living this way."

These threats are sometimes acted upon. In British Columbia two midwives were found guilty of criminal negligence following an infant's death at an attempted home birth. Other midwives have been subject to coroners' inquests or inquiries, and in at least one case serious consideration was given to criminal prosecution following an infant death. In Alberta an established community midwife, Noreen Walker, was charged in 1990 with practising medicine without a licence. In such cases, an infant usually dies or sustains serious injury before a complaint is made. In Walker's case, however, the delivery was successful, and no complaint was registered by the parents (Jiminez 1990). Such legal actions often have a devastating effect on attempts to develop midwifery practice.

Not surprisingly, many midwives have stopped attending home births, partly because of fear of legal action. Lacking legal protection for home birth attendance, and still unwelcome as bona fide practitioners in hospital settings, community midwives have dwindled as a force throughout British Columbia. In 1983 approximately twenty midwives were active in the Lower Mainland; in 1993 only fifteen midwives continued to attend home births. As the birthing population increases, midwives have fallen in numbers. Before discussing the current parodox of legal prohibition in the face of continuing support for women's options in birth, it will be useful to review some historical aspects of laws directed against midwives. Some statutes are quite specific in prohibiting midwifery practice, while at common law charges of criminal negligence are potentially applicable to any citizen. As noted below, however, midwives tend to be the scapegoats for criminal prosecution, unlike more established workers in medicine and nursing.

THE UNLAWFUL PRACTICE
OF MEDICINE:
QUASI-CRIMINAL LAW

Well into the nineteenth century, "midwifery" in North America meant folk or lay midwifery. Licensure was not required, and the extensive apparatus of licensure, legislation and litigation that now characterizes the health professions was very likely unanticipated by indigenous peoples or the early generations of settlers in Canada. With the growth of state authority, however, as well as increased populations and the burgeoning professions of nursing and medicine, childbirth became a site for struggles over who ought to attend births.

As indicated earlier in this book, women's customary assistance of women in childbirth has generally been replaced by a professional monopoly on birth attendance. The traditional birth culture of home remedies and neighbourly assistance – sometimes complemented by a call to a country doctor or local nurse – has been overtaken by modern, professionalized structures of care. These structures were not established without controversy, nor were they impeded by legal protection for many of the folk midwives. In nineteenth-century Ontario, for instance, the right to practise midwifery (independently of physic or surgery) was eventually restricted to medical practitioners (Biggs 1983). The takeover of birth attendance was not so one-dimensional. The right of women to practise midwifery without a licence was recognized in the first legislation passed in Upper Canada. Enforcement was problematic at this time, owing to the limited number of doctors in what was then a predominantly rural region. Nevertheless, section 49 of the Ontario Medical Act held that "it shall not be lawful for any person not registered to practise medicine, surgery or midwifery for hire, gain, or hope of reward, and if any person not registered pursuant to this Act, for hire, gain or hope of reward practises or professes to practise medicine, surgery or midwifery, or advertises to give advice in medicine, surgery, or midwifery, he shall, upon summary conviction thereof before any Justice of the Peace, for every such offence, pay a penalty not exceeding $100 nor less than $25" (see Biggs 1983).

An important qualification was that the alleged illegal practices must encroach on medical practice, and that isolated episodes would not sustain a conviction. Where prosecution under provincial legislation was anticipated, presumably complainants and prosecutors alike would have to contemplate whether these loopholes would affect the likelihood of conviction. As Mr. Justice Garrow indicated:

"The thing practised must, to be illegal, be an invasion of similar things taught and practised by the regular practitioner, otherwise it does not affect the monopoly, and is outside the statute. And it must be practised as the regular practitioner would do it – that is, for gain, and after diagnosis and advice. And it must be more than a mere isolated instance, which is sufficient to prove a 'practice'" (*Re: Medical Act [Ontario]* 1906, 513).

The obligation to prove more than a single act had been upheld in a number of precedents. The conviction of a Toronto midwife under section 49 of the Ontario Medical Act was reversed on appeal. The Appeal Court found that the Crown had not established that the midwife had practised medicine on more than one occasion, and further that she had not always received financial gain through her actions (*R. v. Whelan* 1900). The necessity to prove that financial gain was received and that the illegal practice of medicine occurred repeatedly was crucial in the acquittal of another accused person. The judge in *R. v. Armstrong* (1911) held: "Before an accused person can be convicted of falsely pretending to heal the sick, it is necessary that it be shown that the accused was in the habit of so pretending, or at least that there had been continuous treatment, the principle being the same as practising medicine for gain or hope of reward. An isolated case is not sufficient to secure a conviction." A subsequent decision by Mr. Justice Simmons in *R. v. Cruickshanks* (1914) confirmed that a single act does not constitute the practice of medicine or a trade.

As the state has deliberated over birth-related law, the criterion for an offence has been broadened. In Ontario, the common law rule that "practice" implied repetition of the offending act was altered. A single act was deemed sufficient to establish the practice of medicine. Nevertheless, the prosecution of midwives was not always successful. One criminal conviction of a midwife in the Northwest Territories was quashed on appeal. The court held in *R. v. Rondeau* (1903, 478–83) that section 60 of the Medical Profession Ordinance did not include "midwifery" as a form of practice to be covered along with "medicine" and "surgery." Since section 60 had been composed with reference to the earlier Ontario Medical Act, which prohibited midwifery, medical, and surgical practice by unregistered persons, the court reversed the conviction. The turn-of-the-century *Rondeau* decision was brought forward 90 years later, in the trial of Noreen Walker (discussed below).

Legal prohibitions on the practice of medicine thus served to protect unregistered practitioners, but only to a degree. Lawmakers and judges of the day seemed well aware of the need to facilitate medical practices, and were undoubtedly influenced by the ostensibly progressive spirit of replacing untrained midwives with medical specialists and trained nurses. The courts were not always bloody-minded about who ought to be punished for infractions of the law. Technicalities seemed not to carry the day. In *R. v. Ornavowski* (1941), an orderly accused of practising midwifery and practising medicine, both for "hope of reward," was acquitted on both counts. The court held that the accused orderly had assisted a woman following delivery when no doctor was available to her; that is, he acted in emergency circumstances and did not attempt to charge for his attendance. On the second count, although the accused had on two occasions filled in blank prescription forms, taken patients' temperatures, and given instructions as to treatment, there was no proof of payment or a request for payment by the orderly.

The corollary was also true. Persons practising medicine on more than one occasion and seeking payment for their advice could be convicted (*Provincial Medical Board v. Bond* 1890). The County Court decided in favour of the defendant following a charge under the Medicine and Surgery Act of 1884. The defendant had treated people with plaster and given advice on the use of poultices for people suffering from tumours and cancer. On appeal, however, the initial judgment was reversed: a penalty of $20 for one day's practising and court costs were imposed on the defendant.

About two decades later, in a case heard in Saskatchewan, Mr. Justice Trant declared that the rights of unregistered practitioners are limited and sharply defined. They must not offer diagnosis, give advice, or prescribe medicines (see *R. v. Raffenberg* 1909, 419).

The practice of midwifery in British Columbia has generally been legally protected as the bailiwick of medical practitioners. Section 72 of the British Columbia Medical Practitioners Act stipulated that "(1) a person who practices or offers to practice medicine while not registered or while suspended from practice under this Act commits an offence. (2) For the purposes of and without restricting the generality of subsection (1), a person practices medicine who ... (d) prescribes or administers a treatment or performs surgery, midwifery or an operation or manipulation, or supplies or applies an apparatus or appliance for the cure, treatment or prevention of a human disease, ailment, deformity, defect or injury."

It is important to note that alternative practitioners may be acquitted on charges of the unregistered practice of medicine. In *R. v. Wong* (1979) the court held that the art of acupuncture was not recognized as a branch of medicine by the Alberta College of Physicians and Surgeons. Moreover, acupuncture was not taught in North American medical education. A later conviction of an acupuncturist in British Columbia occurred despite the reasoning in *Wong*. It was held that the defendant had violated the provincial Medical Practitioners Act.

Under section 83 of the Medical Practitioners Act, the minimum penalty for a first offence of practising medicine or midwifery is $100 or imprisonment (section 87). The penalty is $300 or imprisonment for a second conviction, and imprisonment for a third or subsequent conviction. It must be kept in mind that the court has the power to dismiss charges against defendants when the information is insufficient. In one instance where a defendant was charged under the British Columbia Medical Act the information alleging the unlawful practice of medicine was quashed since it failed to set forth the act or acts constituting the alleged offences and failed to name the patients upon whom the defendant was alleged to have unlawfully practised medicine (*R. v. Kripps* 1977).

Under section 73 there are several exceptions to the broad ambit of medical practice set out under section 72. The following practitioners do not practise unlawfully while registered under their respective acts: chiropractors, dentists, naturopaths, optometrists, pharmacists, podiatrists, psychologists, nurses, and dental technicians. Orthotic technicians, physiotherapists, and dieticians may also be exempt from section 72. The legal standing of these practitioners and their self-regulation through professional associations qualifies the purely instrumentalist approach to medicine as an élite profession that is able to monopolize health services. Emergency procedures are permitted under the British Columbia Health Emergency Act. Domestic administration of family remedies is permitted, and religious practitioners "who practise the religious tenets of their church without pretending a knowledge of medicine or surgery" are exempted under section 74 of the act.

The common practice in Canada has been not to charge midwives with practising medicine without a licence unless there has been some tangible damage to the infant or mother in the course of a home birth or during a transfer to hospital following an attempted home birth. Thousands of births have been attended by midwives in Canada in recent years, with very few complaints registered by the parents concerned. In a sense, this testifies to the bond between midwives and their clients, a bond that is clearly not legally recognized. The discretionary power to prosecute midwives for unregistered practice, while rarely exercised, is dormant, and can be brought forward or at least considered.

As a rule, the prosecution of a midwife for unregistered practice would occur only if there was demonstrable harm to the mother or infant. Even so, few such charges had been brought forward through the 1980s in Canada. The prosecution of Noreen Walker is one exception. Walker, a community midwife in Alberta, had practised for over a decade, attending over a thousand births. She was active in supporting women who desired to give birth at home, including those who wished to attempt vaginal birth after a caesarean section. The VBAC option in a home birth is one that is almost universally decried by medical and nursing bodies, but one that has not been proved less safe than hospital-based VBAC (Sufrin-Dusler 1990). Even though the mother, Katherine Charpentier, and the infant were not injured in a VBAC performed at home, Walker was charged as follows: "On or about the 4th day of May, A.D. 1990, at or near Castor, in the Province of Alberta, not being a registered practitioner, [the defendant] did practice or profess to practice medicine, contrary to s. 76 (1) (a) of the Medical Profession Act."

The case was heard before the Alberta provincial court. The Crown called its expert witnesses and other witnesses, ostensibly to call into question the legality of a midwife assisting with VBAC deliveries at home, and perhaps the nature of the defendant's midwifery practice in general. The defence lawyer arranged for expert witnesses to speak in support of the defendant. Moreover, the nature of the defence rested on attempts to challenge the constitutional validity of sections of the Alberta Medical Profession Act. The Notice of Constitutional Question (a notice pursuant to section 4 of the Alberta Bill of Rights) filed by the defence counsel challenges sections 76 and 77 of the act.

(a) Section 76(1) creates an absolute liability offence, or alternatively a strict liability offence, for which imprisonment is a possible sentence, thereby offending s. 7 of the Canadian Charter of Rights and Freedoms [hereinafter "the Charter"].

(b) To the extent that Section 76 creates an offence for the practise of midwifery by a person who is not a "registered practitioner," the section offends s. 7 of the Charter by limiting the life, liberty and security of the person of midwives who are not physicians and surgeons and by limiting the life, liberty and security of the person of women who wish to retain the services of midwives in preparation for and during childbirth.

(c) Section 77 offends s. 11(d) of the Charter by requiring a trier to find that an accused person "practices" contrary to s. 76 where such person does not "practice" but merely does any of the things mentioned in s. 77.

(d) Section 76 and s. 77 offend s. 2(b) of the Charter by purporting to create an offence for professing, or by way of advertising, sign or statement, or by way of claim, makes [sic] certain statements without any requirement of proof of "practise."

(e) Section 76 offends s. 15 of the Charter by discriminating on the basis of sex in that midwives are predominantly women and the section is aimed in part at the suppression of midwifery; or alternatively, by discriminating on the basis of geographic location against midwives who practice midwifery within the limits of a city, town or village having a resident registered practitioner in midwifery therein [notice prepared by the defence lawyer, Simon Renouf].

The notice also alludes to possible violations of part of the Alberta Bill of Rights. The breadth of section 77 (persons who are deemed to practise medicine) is clearly open to interpretation, as is what is meant by the practice of medicine. In the Walker case, VBAC, especially in a home birth situation, was presented by the Crown as a medical procedure. The options of women to give birth in a preferred setting, limitations on doctors' skills or willingness to permit VBACS, and the failure to demonstrate statistically that VBAC women are at greater risk than other women in birth seemed to be part of the defence counsel's efforts to challenge the charge against Walker. Testimony at trial included statements by physicians concerning the inadvisability of attempting a VBAC at home. Other testimony pointed to evidence that VBAC risks have been exaggerated in medical training. Charpentier's obstetrician, Dr. William Young, was alleged to have stripped her membranes without her consent, a procedure not recommended for women seeking a VBAC. Professor Peggy Anne Field, then the president of the Alberta Association of Midwives and a professor of nursing at the University of Alberta, stated that while she would not attend a VBAC at home, "women's choice is paramount" (Williams 1991, 498.) On 5 June 1991, Judge Paul Adilman granted the defence's request for a "directed acquittal," meaning that Walker did not have to take the stand in her own defence, nor did her lawyer, Simon Renouf, need to call his expert witnesses. Judge Adilman noted that while Walker had clearly practised midwifery, "nowhere can I find evidence in this case that Ms. Walker was practising medicine. This was a normal, natural and uncomplicated birth" (see Moysa and Aikenhead 1991).

The legal issues surrounding childbirth become even more complex when one considers the liabilities of parents. In the United States the parents' duty of care has traditionally begun with the birth of the child: there has been no obligation on the part of the mother, for instance, to seek medical assistance prior to the birth. Nevertheless, there appears to be a shift in legal opinion whereby a parent's failure to obtain medical care in circumstances where such care is clearly warranted ought to be culpable (Annas 1977, 180). Parental liability is also an issue with respect to responsibility surrounding midwifery attendance in jursidictions where it is illegal. Klein (1980) stated that the choice of a birth setting – and, by extension, the choice of birth attendants – is the responsibility of the expectant mother. I examined a number of documents (medical histories and midwives' notes made during prenatal visits) that also contained a waiver, signed by the mother (and father, where applicable), which purported to absolve the midwife from liability. Members of the Freemont Birth Collective (1977) linked their philosophy of parental responsibility and decision-making with a non-hierarchial approach to birth management:

Working as a team throughout pregnancy and labor, prospective parents and workers all share in the responsibility for the situation. The woman who is pregnant or in labor, and her support people, are the ones who ultimately make the decisions about what to do, how to proceed. Especially because we're not certified in any way, we're concerned that people analyze their level of comfort working with us. We encourage people to educate themselves as much as possible, consult the statistics we have kept, ask us lots of questions, talk to others who have experienced obstetrical care in other settings, and to make conscious decisions to really think about what they want and to make intelligent judgements.

On another level, legal actions are conventionally brought against the birth attendant, not the expectant mother. This locus of responsibility avoids a direct confrontation with parental rights, and at the same time defines the legal conflict as essentially a dispute pertaining to occupational licensure. Legal protections for unborn children have also been strengthened. In Canada and in other industrialized countries the unborn child has been vested with certain rights. As discussed below, the *Marsh* case in British Columbia held that a child at term – but not yet expelled from the mother – was a person and entitled to protection. As the "human status" of the infant has been explored (Raphael 1975, 67), there appears to have been a rise in litigation in the event of injury or death to fetuses or infants.

The conjunction of medical knowledge and the legal protection of medical practice is best suited to the structural motif of power. The mechanics of touch, palpation, measuring, and viewing of the pregnant woman or fetus have become centred in hospital-based obstetrics, and other forms of practice have been largely excluded. Professional interests are thus protected, even though there has been some erosion of the monopoly status of physicians under quasi-criminal statutes. A related point is that the various medical acts and health disciplines and professions acts serve to enable physicians to practise with little interference. They are enabling of medicine, and stand in stark contrast to their potential repressive application against non-physicians not covered specifically by such acts.

CRIMINAL PROSECUTION OF BIRTH ATTENDANTS

An examination of criminal prosecutions of midwives is crucial to understanding how legal encumbrances have affected midwifery practices, particularly in North America, where midwives' status at law is unsettled. Criminal sanctions can be severe; under Canadian criminal law, the maximum penalty for persons convicted of criminal negligence causing death is imprisonment for life (Bourque 1980). Criminal charges against midwives increased as home births attended by midwives became more prominent in the 1970s and 1980s. Two cases involving midwives charged following infant deaths are reviewed below. We begin, however, with the *Marsh* case, involving an ex-physician charged with criminal negligence in British Columbia.

R. v. Marsh (1979)

In *R. v. Marsh* a spiritual healer (and former doctor) was acquitted on a charge of criminal negligence causing death. The Canadian Criminal Code stipulates that criminal negligence occurs when a person, through commission or omission, shows wanton or reckless disregard for the lives or safety of other persons. The omission or commission must be associated with something that is his or her duty to do. Section 220 (formerly section 203) states that "every one who by criminal negligence causes death to another person is guilty of an indictable offence and is liable to imprisonment for life."

Midwives are quick to point out that Margaret Marsh was not a midwife as such. She had practised as a physician, had not completed a formal course or programme in midwifery, and had not had the benefit of continuity of care with the expectant couple. Marsh had agreed to attend the birth late in the pregnancy, when the couple's midwife was not available.

In the *Marsh* case, the infant's death was attributed to cerebral hemorrhage due to a tear in the tentorium of the skull. This tear was in turn associated with malpresentation of the fetus at term. The legal actions that followed the infant's death were twofold. First, a charge of criminal negligence causing death was laid against Marsh, who had been dropped from the rolls of the College of Physicians and Surgeons of British Columbia. Second, following her acquittal on the above charge, a quasi-criminal charge of practising medicine without a licence in contravention of the British Columbia Medical Practitioners Act was successfully brought against her (McIntyre 1983).

In his reasons for judgment Judge Peter Millward concluded:

Mrs. Marsh first became aware of the unusual and dangerous position of the child when the first foot appeared. By then, the evidence clearly shows it was too late to save the child from the injury that it suffered, or at least on the evidence, it is most unlikely, given the situation, that is a lack of skilled personnel present, the distance in time and space from the hospital, and the lack of any previous arrangements having been made ... On that finding, and with reference to the acts or omissions of Mrs. Marsh from the point in time when the foot first emerged, there cannot be a finding of criminal negligence causing death arising out of those acts or omissions, and accordingly, if any criminal liability is to be attached, it must be found in her acts or omissions prior to that point in time ... a most important point, in my view, is that there is no evidence whatever of any doubt, in the mind of Mrs. Marsh as to the position of the child at that point.

Accordingly, while Mrs. Marsh may have been incompetent, yet I am faced with the evidence of eminent authorities called both by the Crown and by the Defence, to the effect that even the most expert and experienced practitioners do make mistakes from time to time in detecting the position of fetuses in circumstances similar to those which obtained here.

I am faced with that clear evidence and a total lack of any positive evidence of a wanton or willful disregard. I am unable to conclude that any act or omission of Mrs. Marsh, prior to the emergence of the foot, was indeed negligent, and certainly I am unable to conclude that it was criminally negligent.

The *Marsh* case attracted wide media coverage and drew public attention to arguments for and against midwifery. Part of the defence strategy involved raising questions about women's birth experiences in hospital and in other settings. Even in the face of medical opposition to the idea of home births and independent midwifery practice, some medical practitioners are aware of the motivations of women seeking alternative birth care. Dr. Bernd Wittmann, an obstetrician familiar with the midwifery movement in Canada, made the following observations of birthing cultures: "When I arrived 20 years ago in Canada, coming from a European country where midwifery was fully accepted, where physicians were trained by midwives and where in case of an emergency, the physician was forced by law to have a midwife present to help and support the woman. I realize that in North America ... [the situation] was quite opposite. There were deliveries done routinely in the Operating Room, in an OR [operating room]-like environment, on an operation table. The patient's arms and legs were strapped down ... there was a large amount of interference with forceps and episiotomies ... It was quite obvious that women had very negative experiences from their first deliveries. They knew about alternatives ... and decided they were unprepared to go back into this environment, and decided to go for home deliveries" (Interview transcript from *Midwifery and the Law* 1991).

A key point in *Marsh* involved the question whether an infant at term, but not yet expelled from the mother, could be deemed a "person" for the purposes of the Criminal Code. In *Lavoie* (1955), an award for the loss of a child not born alive was denied. In the judgment a human being was described as an entity that has proceeded completely out of the mother's body. Glanville Williams also spoke of the "conditional legal personality" of the unborn child, and said that claims of defendants for negligence injuring unborn children crystallize after the child-plaintiff is born alive (see Samuels 1974, 266).

In *Marsh*, Judge Millward held that a fetus at term, but not yet expelled, could be considered a person for the purposes of the Criminal Code.

The essential nature of the organism, that is the fetus, is not changed by the fact of birth, and to hold that prebirth criminal negligence causing death of a fetus immediately after birth is an indictable offence, while similar negligence causing death immediately before delivery is not criminal, is not a conclusion that accords well with the concept that the state has a duty to protect unborn children and to preserve their opportunities to be born and to enjoy the rights and obligations normally incident to the status of human kind (at 14–15).

While *Marsh* did not directly involve midwives, it did set a modern precedent for the prosecution of an attendant at a home birth. Midwives were faced with the prospect of costly and protracted legal action in the event that an injury (fatal or non-fatal) was brought to the attention of authorities. Within a few years of the *Marsh* case, another prosecution was launched, this time in Halifax, Nova Scotia.

R. v. Carpenter et al. (1983)

In January 1983, Donna Carpenter and Linda Wheeldon, two lay midwives, and Charlene MacLellan, a nurse with postgraduate training in advanced practical obstetrics, were charged with criminal negligence causing bodily harm. The charge followed the home birth of a baby girl and the transfer of the infant to hospital when she did not breathe despite efforts at resuscitation. After determining that the baby had suffered permanent brain damage, a doctor notified the police department and the charge was laid against the three attendants. The charge was amended to criminal negligence causing death in the summer of 1983, a few weeks after the infant's life support system was disconnected. The preliminary inquiry was held over four days in October and November 1983. Judge W.A.D. Gunn decided that the women would not be brought to trial owing to lack of evidence. The charge was dropped at the preliminary hearing prior to the trial. Witnesses at the preliminary inquiry made three key observations: first, the infant suffered a hemorrhage to the portion of her brain that governed breathing; second, the injury was not attributable to the midwives' care; and third, similar injuries had been noted among babies delivered in hospital settings under medical care (Alternative Birth Crisis Coalition 1984).

Cases such as *Carpenter et al.* may be used to highlight the vulnerability of midwives to criminal charges. Criminal cases against physicians and nurses who attend women in labour and delivery are virtually nonexistent in Canada. Peter Leask remarks on this disparity: "When babies die in hospital, sometimes thought is given to civil negligence suits against the hospital and the doctor, and that is of course traumatic for them, but to the best of my knowledge, there is never any thought given to criminal prosecution ... It's treated as a civil matter, as a regulation of the doctor's practice now. I'm completely confident that if midwifery were legalized in this province the same thing would be true about deaths involving midwives. It's the sort of aura of illegality surrounding midwifery that leads to police involvement and the sort of theory that there must be a crime here to prosecute" (*Midwifery and the Law* 1991).

Carpenter et al. was followed a few years later by a case involving two Vancouver midwives following an infant death in Vancouver's west end. This case was much more protracted, and raised many troubling issues concerning the status of the fetus (prior to expulsion) and the appropriateness of charging midwives.

R. v. Sullivan (1986–91)

Two Vancouver midwives were charged with assault, criminal negligence causing death, and other offences following the death of a baby girl on 8 May 1985 in Vancouver. These charges followed the transfer of a mother and unborn child to hospital following an attempted delivery of a shoulder dystocia. This situation, in which the oblique diameter of the pelvic inlet is smaller than the bisacromial diameter, is regarded as an "obstetric emergency" along with other forms of dystocia (see Jensen et al. 1979, 492, 505).

The parents were reported to be supportive of the attending midwives (Sullivan-LeMay Legal Action Fund 1986). Over time, however, there have been reports of the suffering experienced by the mother during labour and after the stillbirth (see Women's Legal Education and Action Fund 1991, 8, 29). Mrs. Voth was later awarded $4,800 through the Criminal Injury Compensation program in British Columbia. The award was given on the basis of "the nature of the injuries sustained and the nature and degree of the pain, suffering, anxiety and inconvenience occasioned by the injuries" (see Workers' Compensation Board 1987, 12). In contrast to other cases involving infant death following transfer to hospital from home, the two midwife-defendants were originally found guilty on the charge of criminal negligence causing death. The midwives were ordered to perform community service and to refrain from attending births, and were placed on probation for two years. Expert witnesses called by the Crown were critical of their management of the birth.

At trial, Judge Godfrey encouraged greater regulation of midwifery practice in British Columbia. Judge Godfrey held that the accused, as childbirth attendants, "were under the legal duty imposed by s. 198 [of the Criminal Code] to use reasonable knowledge, skill and care." The trial judge was critical of the midwifery care, concluding that "the child would have lived had the mother and child been transported to a hospital earlier and had the accused possessed the skills of a medical intern." He concluded that the accuseds' management of the birth "showed a reckless disregard for the life and safety of the child." As discussed below, the judge made a controversial ruling that a child at term, while being born, "was a 'person' within the meaning of s. 203, nothwithstanding that it would not be a 'human being' within the meaning of s. 206." The midwives were also acquitted under section 204 (criminal negligence causing bodily harm), since the mother "had miraculously suffered only bruising."

In March 1987, the Coroner's Court of British Columbia completed a judgment of inquiry into the death of the baby. The coroner held that the death was due to perinatal asphyxia, and that this was an unnatural death. At the time of the judgment, the midwives had already been convicted of criminal negligence causing death. The criminal conviction was reviewed by the British Columbia Court of Appeal, and a conviction for criminal negligence causing bodily harm (to the mother) was substituted for the original conviction of criminal negligence causing death. The decision in this case was controversial in terms of the ruling that for the purposes of section 203, a "full term child in the process of being born [is a] 'person'" until its birth, and also in the decision to substitute a conviction for criminal negligence causing bodily harm (to the mother) in lieu of the original conviction: "The accused had attended as midwives at the birth of a baby but there were complications during the birth and the baby died. (1) The trial judge had concluded that the baby in the circumstances was a 'person' within the meaning of s. 203 but the trial judge erred in that ruling as the baby had never been born alive [*Regina v. Marsh*, 2 CCC (3d) 1 (BC Co. Ct) overruled.] At common law the line of demarcation for a foetus to become a person was the requirement that it be completely extruded from its mother's body and be born alive, and no Parliamentary intention to change that requirement had been established here. The accused could therefore not be convicted under s. 203. (2) It necessarily followed that the child when in the birth canal remained a part of the mother as a matter of law. The trial judge had found that the accused were criminally negligent concerning the baby ... as the trial judge had already determined [that the accused were guilty of criminal negligence causing bodily harm, with respect to the mother], it was appropriate for the court of appeal here to enter that conviction now, and impose the same sentence imposed in respect of the offence under s. 203, [*R. v. Sullivan* (1988), 65 CR (3d) 256 (BCCA)]."

The appellate course was not yet exhausted. The midwives launched an appeal to the Supreme Court of Canada. With leave to appeal granted, the midwives' lawyers, Thomas Berger and Peter Leask, were successful in having the conviction quashed.

This is undoubtedly the most prominent case involving Canadian midwives. The acquittal of LeMay and Sullivan, however, is not a clear victory for midwifery. The trial and appeals tended to focus on the evidence surrounding this particular birth-event, and in the appellate stages attention was redirected to the relatively narrow (in terms of midwifery's status) question of the status of the fetus.

The acquittal of Sullivan and LeMay, the decision in the *Walker* case in Alberta, and the general lack of a modern precedent for the successful prosecution of community midwives in Canada has undoubtedly prompted state authorities to regulate midwives in a less repressive fashion. A case that might have been regarded as a clear violation of midwifery guidelines in some jurisdictions – managing the delivery of twins at home – did not result in the criminal prosecution of a midwife who attended a woman about to have twins. One of the twins was delivered stillborn on 12 April 1990 at the Winnipeg Health Sciences Centre. While it was reported that police were contemplating laying criminal charges against the midwife (Wiecek 1990), the case was instead investigated through the Office of the Chief Medical Examiner in the Manitoba Department of Justice. The cause of death was asphyxia due to compression of the umbilical cord. No judicial recommendations were made (Manitoba Office of the Chief Medical Examiner 1992, 17–18). The case highlighted the differences among the various advocates of midwifery; some favoured the licensing of nurse-midwives, others supported a wider definition of "midwife" that would include community midwives (Paul 1990, Larsen 1991).

INQUESTS INTO INFANT DEATHS

Although criminal charges are rarely brought against midwives in Canada, midwives who are charged are unlikely to be convicted. Another legal route, one not connected with the guilt-innocence dichotomy of adversarial criminal actions, is to proceed with a provincial coroner's hearing. Inquests involve recommendations by a jury of citizens; inquiries are conducted by the Coroner's Office without convening a jury.

The death of Daniel McLaughlin-Harris in October 1984 in Toronto, Ontario, was followed by a provincial inquest in 1985. Two midwives had attended the mother in labour at a Toronto Island residence. The baby was born asphyxiated, and was transported to the Hospital for Sick Children by one of the midwives. The inquest dealt with the causes of the infant's death and the viability of midwifery as an independent profession. The jury concluded that the death was attributable to oxygen deprivation, and that the death could have been prevented had the mother been transported to hospital at an earlier stage. The need for better monitoring of the infant's heartbeat and the importance of more "sophisticated" resuscitation equipment was also noted by the jury (Report of the Ontario Task Force 1987, 31).

The coroner's jury made several recommendations to alter the status of midwifery in Ontario. First, it recommended that the Ontario Health Disciplines Act be rewritten to specify what constitutes midwifery practice, and that strict penalties for illegal practice be imposed for practice outside the Act. Second, midwifery should be undertaken as a specialty practice under the jurisdiction of the College of Nurses of Ontario; after five years, an independent college of midwives should be established. Third, midwifery training should conform to the international standards established by the International Federation of Obstetricians and Gynecologists and the International Confederation of Midwives (Burtch 1992, 168). To practise, a person would require at least two years' midwifery training and a year of general nursing. Fourth, licensed midwives should be given hospital privileges in maternity wards. Fifth, Ontario Health Insurance Plan coverage should be available for midwives' services and malpractice insurance should be compulsory. Sixth, birthing centres should be established in hospitals. Seventh, the option of home birth attendance should be available within the Ontario health care system. Finally, the College of Physicians and Surgeons should establish safety standards for home births, and doctors should be free from censure by their colleagues if they attend home births (Besheraw 1985, 11).

The Coroner's Office in Burnaby, British Columbia, has also been involved in cases involving midwife-assisted births. In addition to *Sullivan and LeMay* (discussed above), two other cases received considerable publicity. A coroner's inquiry in 1986 concluded that the responsibility for some infant deaths associated with midwives' attendance at attempted home births fell on the government for its failure to resolve a "state of uncertainty" surrounding midwifery and home birth. Chief Coroner Robert Galbraith (since retired) held that the midwife (Gale Gray) had contacted the back-up physician when she noted a drop in fetal heartrate. The midwife arranged for the mother to be transported to hospital. Despite rescuscitation efforts by hospital staff, the infant (baby McLean) was pronounced dead. It is significant that the parents of the stillborn baby supported and continue to support the midwife (see *Midwifery and the Law* 1991). Both parents also commented on the difficulties in actually making the transition from home to hospital, where the midwife was treated as an outsider rather than the person who "knew most about the birth" (*Midwifery and the Law* 1991). The parents also noted that the formal proceedings of the coroner's inquiry, with legal representation, publicity, and so forth, militated against their being able to maintain regular contact with the midwife after the death and before the inquiry.

The second case, which involved the death of an infant (baby Bellingrath) on 13 May 1985, was complicated by the parents' criticism of the attending midwife. As noted earlier, it is rare for parents not to support midwives even in tragedies associated with home births. In this case, the British Columbia Coroner's Service ordered an autopsy when it was known that the midwife had been involved prior to the mother's caesarean section at Grace Hospital. The autopsy was ordered "in light of the current controversy surrounding the illegal practice of midwifery in the province of British Columbia" (*Verdict*, Coroner's Court of British Columbia 1988).

This case generated considerable activity in the Coroner's Office, the major crimes unit of the Vancouver City Police, and even in the Supreme Court of British Columbia. (In 1987 the court held that once the filing of the judgment of inquiry had been made, by law the coroner could not legitimately rehear the case or order an inquest.) In 1986 information was received that the attorney-general would not recommend criminal prosecution of the midwife or the back-up physician. Nevertheless, in February 1988, the attorney-general ordered an inquest.

Seventeen witnesses appeared at the inquest. They included the mother and father of the deceased child, the attending midwife, a consulting midwife, several physicians, and a nurse from Grace Hospital, among others. Twenty-two exhibits were filed. The verdict of the coroner's inquest was that the baby's death was accidental and due to asphyxia.

It was recommended that midwifery should be legalized and midwives granted "autonomous professional status" in cases of low-risk obstetrics. It was further recommended that a task force be set up to investigate the midwifery situation in British Columbia and that midwives have independent powers to admit women to hospital. The establishment of a college of midwives was also recommended to create and enforce standards of discipline, education, practice, and certification. It was also suggested that midwives be integrated into the provincial health care system.

Other recommendations were directed to the Midwives' Association of British Columbia, including that improvements be made in providing labour records and prenatal documentation when mothers are transferred to hospital. Concern was expressed over the need for guidelines for monitoring fetal heartbeat and vital signs, and the importance of the midwife alerting hospital staff to the impending arrival at hospital. Recommendations to Grace Hospital included synchronization of clocks throughout the hospital (to assist in the sequencing of events), a review of admission procedures, and a recommendation that staff "be receptive to incoming phone calls from midwives who are informing of pending arrival and condition of mother" (Coroner's Court of British Columbia 1988). Kaufman (1989) viewed the inquest recommendations as demonstrating "clear and unequivocal support for recognition of midwifery."

The abstract notion that the state, through the law, acts in a neutral way to resolve disputes and to make recommendations seems quite distant from the effects of such hearings on the people concerned. Peter Leask has drawn attention to the emotional costs of legal proceedings; financial costs are also a major factor for midwives and their supporters: "I don't know any midwife who's making anything approaching a decent living from being a midwife, and any legal case instantly will cost the equivalent of years of income ... if we're talking about a prosecution, many, many years of income, [and] even for something like an inquiry or inquest, multiple years of income" (Peter Leask, quoted in *Midwifery and the Law* 1991).

There are cases, such as Noreen Walker's in Alberta, where former clients, other supporters, and even chiropractors contribute to a substantial defence fund (approximately $20,000, as of 1991) for the midwife. Lawyers may also represent the midwife at a reduced rate, or, as in Walker's case, on a pro bono basis. In fact, Walker's lawyer, Simon Renouf, had involved himself in earlier disputes, including the 1982 nurses' strike in Alberta, where he was the union director of the United Nurses of Alberta. The point remains, however, that most midwives (Growe 1991, 143) lack the legal expertise and financial resources to cope easily with formal proceedings. Another point arising from the coroner's hearings into midwifery is that all hearings have recommended the legalization of midwifery, and the individuals making recommendations have been attentive to the midwives' insistence on a sphere of practice distinct from medicine or nursing.

CRIMINAL NEGLIGENCE AND PHYSICIANS

Canadian case law reveals few instances in which charges of criminal negligence causing death have been brought against doctors attending births. (There are cases involving therapeutic abortions, most notably those involving Henry Morgentaler [Morton 1993].) In *Simard* (1964) the conviction of a physician for criminal negligence was quashed on appeal to the Quebec Court of Queen's Bench. A newborn child had died of a cerebral hemorrhage a few days following delivery by forceps. Nevertheless, the appeal judges clearly felt that the facts of the case did not warrant the jury's finding of guilt. Those facts included the mother's wish not to give birth in a hospital but rather at a clinic, her failure to follow Dr. Simard's suggestion of an X-ray for suspected cephalopelvic disproportion, and her departure from the birth setting against the doctor's advice.

The court also accepted expert testimony vindicating the use of chloroform and forceps and rejected contrary opinion on this point.

The *Rogers* (1968) case involved an ex-physician and practising naturopath, Dr. Everly Rogers. Dr. Rogers was charged with criminal negligence causing death. His patient, a two-year old boy, Leonidis Demosten, suffered from dermatitis and was put on a very low protein diet in April 1966. The boy lost weight and died in hospital in June 1966 as a result of gross malnutrition. In dismissing an appeal by the accused, the principle of competency required by law was reaffirmed: "In enacting s. 187 [of the Criminal Code] Parliament has imposed a legal duty upon every one who undertakes to administer medical treatment. Included in that legal duty is to have 'reasonable knowledge' in doing so. The essence of that 'reasonable knowledge' was that a physician (which Rogers was) should have foreseen the harmful consequences of depriving the child of proteins and calories in the circumstances. Regardless of his personal theories, Rogers was under a duty to have that foresight. It was, therefore, irrelevant for the jury to consider Rogers' own belief that his diet was a beneficial treatment" (at 299). Mr. Justice Nathan Nemetz concluded as follows: "It was open to the jury here, on the evidence before them, to consider whether Rogers, in knowing the deteriorating condition of this child, yet obstinately continuing the administration of a diet based on his personal theory of medical treatment, was criminally negligent within the meaning of the *Criminal Code* of Canada. Since, in my opinion, no error has been shown to exist in the charge, I would dismiss the appeal" (at 301).

Physicians are subject to malpractice actions and peer review, but are rarely brought into the criminal courts for childbirth-related practice. Community midwives are aware that they are vulnerable to possible criminal investigation and prosecution arising from home birth attendance, and many midwives indicated that this differential application of the criminal law is unjust. A community midwife interviewed in Vancouver in 1985 put this bluntly in 1985: "Hospital staff tend to perpetrate a number of offences against people, things that are negligent, even criminally negligent, against patients. But they get away with it because they are protected by the system." Despite the argument that up to a third of perinatal deaths in hospital are preventable, criminal actions do not ensue against established practitioners.

CIVIL SUITS AGAINST BIRTH ATTENDANTS

There are fewer malpractice suits against physicians (on a per capita basis) in Canada than in the United States. While 20,000 malpractice suits were launched in the United States in one year, only 200 to 300 were initiated in Canada (Coburn 1980, 14). MacIsaac (1976, 204), using data from the Canadian Medical Protective Association, reported that between 1966 and 1970 the number of monetary settlements against its members averaged 18 per year; in 1971, 22 monetary settlements resulted from 131 writs against its members.

In a 1981 case concerning the death from hypoxia of an infant in a Vancouver hospital, the Supreme Court of British Columbia ordered payment of unspecified damages to the family. The nursing care afforded the mother was deemed to have fallen below the expected standard of care, and the attending physician failed to establish the progress of labour before prescribing painkillers. Lack of suctioning equipment in the emergency bundle and the absence of attending staff for thirty minutes while the plaintiff was in labour were other factors cited in the decision (Anonymous 1981).

Coburn (1980) suggests that judges in Canada are generally sympathetic to physicians because of a common status. This notion of class affinity is developed further with respect to the British judiciary and the Canadian judiciary (Miliband 1973; Olsen 1980). At the same time, there is little evidence of civil suits launched against community midwives by their clients. It is noteworthy, however, that as American nurse-midwives have become established as professionals in hospital and clinic settings, they are increasingly subject to malpractice actions (Sinquefield 1983).

RECONSIDERING LAW AND SOCIAL MOVEMENTS

There is ample evidence that dominant groups invoke their powers to exclude competing groups. While there are limits to its powers (Giddens 1982), the state is central to these exclusory attempts. It has the power to criminalize behaviour, to adjudicate civil matters, and to direct its financial resources to specific groups. Ursel (1988) regards the state as a central force in maintaining patriarchal relations and assisting in the transition from familial patriarchy to social patriarchy. At this point I turn to the patriarchal elements of obstetrical practice, and to an examination of how community midwifery presents a challenge to these practices. Hospital-based birth attendance is directed by physicians; less commonly, responsibility may be delegated to nursing personnel. Physicians' incomes remain well above the average incomes of other North Americans; midwives' incomes are markedly lower than average, especially community midwives. Concern has also been expressed over patriarchy in law. The term is used here to mean "a specific organization of the family and society, in which heads of families [control] not only the reproductive labor, but also the production of all family members" (see Gordon and Hunter 1977–8, 12). Ursel (1988, 108) defines patriarchy as "a system or set of social relations that operates to control reproduction through the control of women both in their reproductive and productive labour."

Community midwifery in British Columbia and other regions is a concrete instance of resistance to medical dominance in the management of childbirth and the provision of prenatal and postnatal care. As noted above, attempts to use the courts to prosecute midwives under the Criminal Code have not always been successful. Even quasi-judicial hearings such as coroners' inquests do not automatically reinforce the authority of medical control over birth: two recent coroners' inquiries in Ontario recommended the legal recognition of midwives and the establishment of a provincial school of midwifery.

Legal struggles and the continuing dominance of physicians' authority in Canadian maternity care touch directly on the criticism of western legal ideology for the adherence to notions of a formal, abstract equality of citizens despite substantive inequalities before the law (Burtch 1992). Similarly, there have been serious criticisms of the ways in which pluralist theories of the state fall short, with policies of intolerance and repression evident in Canada and elsewhere (Knutilla 1992; McRae 1979). Some socialist writers, while acknowledging the role of law in perpetuating inequality, have favoured the *use* of law as a form of political struggle (Sumner 1981; Beirne and Sharlet 1980; Fine 1984). In the health-care sector, some have favoured "democratic relativism" as a means of protecting unorthodox forms of medicine and healing, thereby permitting comparisons of the various forms of health care (Feyerabend 1980). These struggles should not overshadow the continuing protection of professional attendance and medical dominance in Canada and elsewhere.

A key consideration is to determine when midwifery practice is demonstrably as safe as (or safer than) conventional physician-managed deliveries, and when it may be more hazardous. This issue is addressed directly in chapter five. A related point concerns the role of the state in promoting or containing midwifery initiatives. Laws that largely buttress the professional dominance of obstetricians and general practitioners are one case in point. By the state's vesting policing powers with the medical colleges, and through the occasional prosecution of alternative practitioners, the implementation of safe, pluralistic maternity care services remains greatly constrained.

Much of the literature concerning midwifery emphasises the role of parental choices in childbirth. This emphasis is seen as complementary to professional concerns about standards of care; well-informed parents should be able to choose from a variety of birth options without compromising their health or that of their children. For many, the existing law in Canada does not adequately recognize the issue of parental rights in childbirth. Peter Leask, a Vancouver-based lawyer, favours a legal model that parallels European systems, including respect for parents' choices: "There's no doubt in my mind that for those who want to change the law, the direction to go is the European model where written into the statutes that govern birth is a right of parents to choose, and a corresponding protection for birth attendants so that if parents make a choice which is not recommended, if the attendant has conscientiously given the safest advice and the parents choose something else, the attendant can still give as much help as possible in whatever birthing choice the parents have made. Here in B.C., in effect we have the opposite situation. The only situation where doctors can assist parents to give birth is a hospital, and any parent who doesen't choose that option has to have either no attendant or an illegal attendant, a situation *everyone* knows is unsafe" (quoted in *Midwifery and the Law* 1991).

The obstetrical system in Holland is frequently presented as an example of a system that promotes parental choices in birth, together with a record of maternal and infant safety. Anderson (1986, 13–14) attributes the success of the Dutch system to three factors: the establishment of highly trained midwives as "primary caregivers," clear guidelines for referral of clients seeking home births, and thorough post-partum care by maternity-aid nurses. This system of referral and training is coupled with a culture that promotes birthing choices. Lee Saxell, a community midwife who discontinued practice following a coroner's inquest, has remained active with the midwifery movement in Canada. She notes that Dutch women continue to use a variety of birthplaces, and that their culture supports childbirth. Birth is "accepted into the culture. Almost every child will be in a house where someone has given birth, or a neighbour who's just given birth and they can see a brand newborn baby. Children are very often at the births if they're family members ... [while some Canadian women are reluctant to go to hospital, for fear of unnecessary intervention] you don't see that so much in Holland where they're not afraid to go in; they would just prefer to be at home. It's more comfortable and it's perfectly normal. No one's told them that it's radical or dangerous. It's accepted into the culture. There are images of birth and pregnant women all over Holland ... it's just more commonplace to see those sorts of images of pregnant women as being a normal part of the culture than it is here in North America" (*Midwifery and the Law* 1991). This coherent system contrasts with the malintegrated legal interventions that have characterized midwifery trials and inquiries in Canada. These interventions have to date imposed considerable costs on midwives, without building on recommendations that the legal practice of midwifery be established and promoted.

The net effect of the threat of criminal prosecution or a coroner's investigation has been that many senior community midwives have stopped attending home births. They cite costs, publicity, and uncertainty as factors that discourage their practice. Peter Leask notes that although community midwives manifest more caring for people and their income "does not approach a decent standard of living," they are faced with legal costs equivalent to "many, many years of income" if there is criminal prosecution (*Midwifery and the Law* 1991). In general, low incomes have been the standard for community midwives in Canada (Barrington, 1985).

In Lee Saxell's case, criminal charges were not laid, although a coroner's inquest was called following an infant's death after an attempted home birth: "Even though every midwife knows statistically that eventually it's going to happen, still it was devastating to me, and I was really emotionally distraught by the whole thing. I continued practising, and then when the death went to inquest three years later and I went through that whole process which was extremely lengthy because of the time that it took me to prepare and then recover, then I felt that I couldn't practice again because I couldn't risk that again. It's a sort of thing that you'd never want to do more than once. Anyone I know who has been through it, any other midwife in Canada feels the same way" (*Midwifery and the Law* 1991).

The lack of legal recognition has encouraged midwives to leave practice, and it has had a chilling effect on the recruitment of new midwives. This means that in contrast to other, more recognized professions, such as nursing and medicine, new cohorts of midwives are not being produced regularly in Canada. The "trials of labour" also serve to drain the limited funds of groups such as the Midwives Association of British Columbia; money that was raised in support of midwifery practice and education is diverted to legal costs. Legal defence funds are usually raised by soliciting former clients of midwives and by sponsoring gaming activities (such as casino benefits) in British Columbia (Burtch, 1987).

The "legalization of politics" (Mandel 1989) poses considerable costs for midwives, and deflects legal discourse away from issues such as parental choice, and the integration of midwifery into Canadian health care. Midwives have lobbied for the power to regulate their profession. A College of Midwives could enable midwives to establish guidelines for the safe management of labour and birth and to review instances where such management was called into question. Not all midwives favour such a proposal. Self-regulated professions are rarely independent, and midwives would very likely be controlled to some extent by provincial health officials. It is also not clear if medical and nursing associations would support the proposal for a separate College of Midwives in any Canadian province. Midwives themselves have expressed concern over the ways in which midwifery practice could be restricted as guidelines became more conservative, and penalties (fines, suspensions, loss of a licence) became established.

Raymond DeVries (1985) examined how violations of regulatory law by American midwives raise serious questions about the value of legal regulation of practice. He noted cases in which "lay" midwives were arrested and required to post substantial bonds for bail ($25,000 in the case of a California midwife arrested in 1970; murder charges were dropped only after preliminary hearings) and cases in which other forms of disciplinary action were taken. Subject to a licensing law, midwives' practices are not reviewed by peers alone, but by "a legal code that defines acceptable and unacceptable behavior" (DeVries 1985, 120). Ironically, where midwives are not subject to regulatory laws, several factors can operate in their favour. These include the rarity of charges being brought by clients against midwives, the reluctance of clients to testify against midwives, the generation of positive publicity concerning alternative birth practices, the mobilization of financial and other support from other midwives, and a tradition of "hesitancy on the part of the courts to penalize unlicensed midwives" (DeVries 1985, 121).

The discipline of licensed midwives is another matter. Once licensed, midwives are subject to the scrutiny of medical personnel. In two cases in Arizona, midwives were either suspended from practice or had their licences revoked. One case involved assistance at a diagnosed breech birth, the other a decison to let the parents grieve the baby's death (when fetal heart tones could not be detected) instead of requesting medical assistance immediately. Both actions were in violation of the state law regulating midwifery practice. Midwives in Arizona are not only subject to complaints by physicians about conduct that may be inappropriate or illegal. They are also integrated into a health network, so that they must file detailed reports with the state Department of Health Services. These reports can be reviewed at any time. DeVries draws special attention to the lack of media coverage of the Arizona cases. Significantly, "midwife organizations and alternative birth groups did not rally to the support of the accused" (DeVries 1985, 131).

DeVries takes a cautious approach to the value of licensing midwives. He points out that licensing schemes tend to remove opportunities for "consumer evaluation" of practitioners, while medical associations and state officials become more involved in reviewing and disciplining midwives for breaches of licensing regulations. Legalization may thus have an untoward effect on the very midwives who seek legal status, and on their clientele.

DeVries's work highlights the dilemma of recourse to state law in regulating parental choices and midwifery practice. As we have seen, the use of repressive law, such as criminal prosecution, has traditionally not resulted in conviction of unlicensed midwives, and legal costs are invariably high. The adversarial effect of such actions can widen the gulf between midwives and physicians. But DeVries (1985, 136–7) holds that where licensing is established, midwives subject to legal codes face loss of the right to practise midwifery and possibly the loss or suspension of a nursing licence. The once-blurred legal status of midwives practising outside the system is sharpened by legalization, but in a manner that retains an edge of punitiveness. Gaskin (1988, 56) reinforces DeVries's argument, noting that restrictions on certain practices – such as midwives' being prohibited from administering drugs to stop hemorrhaging – may lead midwives to conceal certain aspects of birth care.

It has also been pointed out that legalization in itself does not guarantee adequate midwifery services. Midwifery can be established, certainly, but it can also be whittled away or removed. Gaskin (1988, 56) cites the case of a Florida law allowing direct-entry midwifery. The law was passed following years of lobbying by the Florida Midwives Association; however, a counter-lobby of Florida physicians succeeded in reversing the direct-entry law. Midwives who had completed direct-entry training could continue practising, but to other aspirants the door was closed. Even in European countries where midwifery is well established, recent policies have led to fragmented obstetrical care. This fragmentation clearly undermines the continuity of care that midwives prize. Vicki Van Wagner (1984, 1991) notes that the role of the midwife as an advocate for women is compromised by greater recourse to technology ("machine-minding"), rising rates of caesarean sections, and other measures that erode the "close personal social support" traditionally provided by midwives.

The reappearance of community-based, independent midwifery practice in Canada in the mid-1970s challenged the medicalization of childbirth. As a countercultural movement in Canada and elsewhere, midwifery offered an alternative to hospital-based, professionally directed birth management. The appropriation of childbirth by the (predominantly male) medical profession, and the cultural definition of women as incapable of managing birth, were strongly contested in theory and practice by midwives. Reversing the notion of midwives as anachronistic, midwives have sought to argue for midwifery as a highly skilled and sensitive role (Flint, 1986). This struggle focuses not only on the modern takeover of obstetrics by medical and nursing specialists, but on a legacy of repression of alternative healers in Europe and North America, including midwives and herbalists (Ben-Yehuda, 1980; Ehrenreich and English, 1973).

The nature of Canadian midwifery has been transformed in recent years. On the one hand, midwifery has been supported on the international level. The 1993 Congress of the International Confederation of Midwives was held in Vancouver (the first time the congress has been convened in Canada), and British Columbia midwives have completed clinical placements outside Canada (in Holland, Germany, the United States, Jamaica, and England). Community midwifery still exists in British Columbia and other Canadian provinces, but such community-based practice is not well integrated with the established health-care system of billing under medical insurance plans, hospital privileges for practising midwives, and malpractice insurance coverage. In British Columbia some community midwives fear prosecution and have abandoned their practices. The midwifery project at the Grace Hospital has not been expanded to match requests for such midwifery attendance. The midwifery debate in Canada may well founder on a co-opted version of midwifery that would place constraints on autonomous midwifery as it was practised in the 1970s and 1980s. These constraints include mandatory liability insurance, conservative guidelines for practice, no clear official commitment to encouraging out-of-hospital births, and mandatory supervision by physicians of midwives during patients' labour and delivery.

The development of midwifery policy in Canada has been largely arrested through government failure (aside from Ontario and Alberta) to implement midwifery services despite recommendations from numerous quarters, sensationalized media accounts of medical crises at home births, a pervasive ideology of physician dominance of childbirth, and the chilling effect of legal interventions. These trials of midwifery reflect deep contradictions in the construction of women's power (as workers and throughout pregnancy), and the power of criminal and quasi-criminal laws in securing social ordering.

The midwifery movement has implications for state theory: for example, it demonstrates ways in which social movements can gain greater access to resources and in some cases to achieve greater legal recognition. Midwifery may possess greater leverage than some other social movements in that it is potentially a source of legitimacy for existing governments. Implementation of midwifery would seem to vindicate the dominant ideology of liberalism, especially in terms of pluralistic choice of services and responsiveness of the legislature and health-related government services. Not surprisingly, midwifery has been mooted as a cost-saving initiative that would reduce unnecessary surgery, for instance, and in so doing would reduce morbidity (injury) to mothers and newborns (Ontario Task Force 1987, 2).

Midwifery nevertheless must face the consequences of cutbacks in certain services (Dobbin 1990). Further, midwives must resist the tendency to find a Machiavelli behind every government initiative. The provision of safe, secure environments for birth is arguably an initiative that is properly fostered by governments. The importance of infant safety is acknowledged by Canadian midwives. The Canadian midwifery movement is concerned not only with the implementation of safe maternity and infant services in Canada, but also with the reduction of infant and maternal mortality in the developing world. On the world scale, given that 99 per cent of women who die from childbirth-related complications are from the developing world, increased government support for safety worldwide would seem very valuable (see Hsia 1991, 85). The scale of maternal mortality in the developing world is evident in Dr. Malcolm Potts's vivid illustration: "Every four hours, day in, day out, a jumbo jet crashes and all on board are killed. The 250 passengers are all women, most in the prime of life, some still in their teens. They are all either pregnant or recently delivered of a baby. Most of them have growing children at home, and families that depend on them" (cited in Maine 1986, 175). The World Health Organization (who) estimated that nearly 13 million children aged five years and under died in 1990. One-third of those children died within a month of their births (Report of the Director General 1991, 2). The litmus test of the efficacy of such government roles, however, is whether actions by authorities take on a repressive, obstructive character, or whether they actively promote maternal and infant wellbeing in the developing world and elsewhere.

The midwifery movement also poses a challenge to the hegemonic status of medicine. The hegemonic ideology of woman and birth – the notion that birth is a medical event and that women and fetuses must be continually monitored by new technology, and the general eclipse of community bonds as medical and legal experts occupy the terrain of birth – has also been challenged. But the state use of legal force has clearly not been successful in establishing social policies *against* midwives. Time and again in trials and inquests authorities in Canada and elsewhere have been advised of the viability of midwifery, and the unfortunate illegal or alegal status of midwives.

It is also significant that the midwifery movement incorporates traditional values of collective life, along with what Melucci (1978, 205) calls "fresh hypotheses." Dramatized by the peace and environmental movements, and also applicable to the midwifery movement, is the link between private and public spheres. In these contemporary social movements there is "a complementarity between private life, in which new meanings are directly produced and experienced, and publicly expressed commitments. Living differently and changing society are seen as complementary ... One does not live to be a militant. Instead, one lives, and that is why from time to time one can be a public militant" (Melucci 1988, 206).

The reappearance of a community-based, independent midwifery practice in British Columbia in 1975 was followed by a series of events that have transformed the nature of the original movement. Begun as a collective initiative with a primary emphasis on the safety of mothers and neonates, great importance was placed on supporting women seeking birth outside hospital and without recourse to unnecessary medical interventions, including caesarean section, forceps delivery, induction of labour, episiotomy, and analgesia and anaesthesia. The politics of midwifery as a countercultural movement were articulated in Raven Lang's *Birth Book* and Ina May Gaskin's *Spiritual Midwifery*, and in a wider set of practices and writings surrounding women's health care. The appropriation of childbirth by the predominantly male medical profession and the cultural definition of women as incapable of managing birth were strongly contested by midwives.

The human agency – action and consciousness – of British Columbia midwives has been altered in contradictory ways. Other midwifery organizations, most notably in Ontario, have persisted in working toward independent practice, legally recognized and supported through such government auspices as post-secondary education. For Canadian midwives, playing host to the 1993 Congress of the International Confederation of Midwives in Vancouver was a major coup. Another accomplishment was the development of the Vancouver-based Midwifery School. Accredited by the Washington State Department of Health, the school graduated twenty-eight students and has established several preceptorships (clinical placements) internationally. The school ceased operation because of limited enrolment, which was in turn linked with the lack of a legal status for trained midwives in the province. Finally, coroners' inquests and inquiries have in general regarded midwifery care favourably, and have recommended the legal recognition of qualified midwives.

Another phenomenon is the growing effort to establish coalitions among midwives. The *realpolitik* of professional resistance and limited resources among pro-midwifery groups has led to the formation of broader alliances. In British Columbia, for example, the Midwives Association has established working relationships with the Western Midwives Association, the Midwifery Task Force, the Midwives Association of North America, and the International Confederation of Midwives, and has maintained contact with provincial government representatives (such as officials of the Ministry of Health), the Registered Nurses' Association of British Columbia, and the British Columbia Medical Association, among others. Gaskin notes a growing interest in midwifery among u.s. women, adding that the most effective strategy for associations favourable to midwifery is to enter into coalitions. The Midwives Alliance of North America (MANA) is one example of solidarity among different kinds of midwives. Such solidarity holds the promise of extending beyond practising midwives and numerous associations that promote midwifery care, to society at large (Gaskin 1988, 59–60). Ehrenreich and English (cited in Edwards and Waldorf 1984, 195) envision a wider consciousness of birthing and childcare, such that those activities are not left to the responsibility of individual women, but recast as a "transcendent public priority."

A more cooperative model of midwifery seeks the support of government officials and medical and nursing associations, and aims for the legalization of midwifery as a semi-autonomous profession. This cooperative model, as it stands, undermines certain principles of the midwifery movement, especially the desirability of independent midwifery. Nonetheless, it would allow midwives to assess their practices, to assist one another, to respect women's wishes for intimacy and safety, and to work without routine medical supervision or subordination within the hierarchy of hospital care.

One concern is that midwifery will be absorbed within a nurse-midwifery model. A professional model would very likely include mandatory liability insurance, adherence to guidelines of practice, statutory recording and reporting policies (to be reviewed by government), and no clear commitment to respecting out-of-hospital births. This rather sinister picture of state surveillance and discipline is not the final word, however. Midwives have generally favoured legal status, but only if midwifery is seen as standing apart from medical and nursing colleges. The illegal or alegal status of midwives in Canada is clearly not tenable for most midwives, given the attrition rate in recent years and the difficulties experienced by midwives working without colleagial support or other resources (Benoit 1988, 1991). An auxiliary status for midwives is equally untenable. Professionalized midwifery would link Canadian midwives more directly with midwives worldwide, through such organizations as the International Confederation of Midwives.

CONCLUSION

In British Columbia, midwifery policy has been formulated, or deferred, by contrasting midwife-based initiatives against policy declarations of more dominant groupings, notably state officials, and spokespersons for the medical association and the registered nurses' association. It is suggested that while there is some autonomy on the part of these groupings with respect to positions on midwifery practice, the midwifery initiative has retained a sense of integrity (in its demands and practices) without substantially altering the power structure of obstetrics and state control over women's health care. Its achievements to date have involved changes in birthing practices in hospital and a legacy of re-establishing, albeit for a very short time, a range of birthing options, including midwife-attended home birth.

While there is resistance to full implementation of midwifery care in many Canadian jurisdictions, the recommendations of international associations lend considerable support to the movement for qualified midwifery services. The International Confederation of Midwives, for example, has supported the implementation of midwifery in Canada. The World Health Organization (1987) said that "the training of professional midwives or birth attendants should be promoted. Care during normal pregnancy and birth, and following birth should be the duty of this profession."

These developments in midwifery advocacy and practice underline the importance of human agency in shaping culture. As the conflicting evidence is weighed, it is clear that there are no telling arguments against the implementation of midwifery services as part of Canadian social policy. Opponents of midwifery seem to keep midwives in the backcourt (through expensive litigation and a litany of what are, in my view, fallacious arguments concerning skills, women's preferences in childbirth, and costs of establishing midwifery training). Midwives are moving to the forecourt, however, and have access to international support via the ICM and a growing research base made up of professional journals such as *Midwifery* and the

Journal of Nurse-Midwifery, the Midwives Information and Resource Services (MIDIRS), and ongoing work by Page, Tew, Flint, Kitzinger, Rothman, Benoit, and others.

In many other jurisdictions, midwives' efforts for recognition indeed reflect "inter-professional rivalries" (Donnison, 1977). Nevertheless, there is a sense that the dominant approach in law and social policy in Canada is very much out of touch. The examples of Ontario and Quebec, the two most populous provinces in Canada, as they move toward the implementation of midwifery very likely signals a greater integration of midwives in all aspects of birth care. The political will of government officials, court officials, legislators, and the medical and nursing professions is likely to be decisive in positioning midwives. Legal struggles to re-establish parental rights and restore a sense of community of women in childbirth are necessary to achieve innovations in birthcare. As Carol Smart (1989) has cautioned, however, it is crucial that we recognize that new forms of legal control may create substantial gaps between what women seek by way of freedoms and what is offered to them in policies.

CHAPTER SIX

Moving into Midwifery: Paradoxes of Legalization

INTRODUCTION

A generation ago, the twin issues of medicalization of birth and professional control of women's reproductive capacity brought into focus the ways in which childbirth was managed. For critics of obstetrical procedures, medicalized births reflected the (mis)management of birth. Recourse to medicated birth and rising rates of caesarean sections, episiotomies, perineal shaves, forceps deliveries, and induction of labour no longer were characterized as "progressive" birthing practices. As part of an effort to humanize obstetrics and allow for birthing situations tailored to women's needs, the movement has lobbied for the legal recognition of midwifery as a self-governing profession. Legalization would herald an end to the criminal trials used to examine midwifery practice, and would establish midwives as expert practitioners in the management of uncomplicated births. Specifically, many supporters of midwifery wish to obtain not only legal status for the midwife, but a degree of autonomy in practice. Midwifery controlled by other professionals – notably physicians or nurses – would, for these advocates, be midwifery in name only. The gap between fully fledged midwifery services and compromised services is evident for midwives in various countries (see Kitzinger 1988).

Midwifery in North America has met with a mixture of support and resistance. This has led to the current "state of uncertainty" surrounding midwifery observed by the former chief coroner of British Columbia, Robert Galbraith. The prosecution of midwives for criminal negligence and the calling of coroners' inquiries and inquests do little to alleviate this state of uncertainty. Midwives seek to assert their own hegemonic status as experts in the management of normal obstetrics. This role would stand apart from obstetrical nursing, general medical practice, and specialty obstetrics. Self-regulation through a college of midwives would be sought. Midwifery, as envisioned by many midwives, would require a greater recognition of parental rights, and continuity of care for expectant mothers through pregnancy, labour, and delivery and into the postpartum period. While the midwifery movement has secured international recognition in recent years, there has been a pattern of midwives leaving independent practice. In British Columbia this usually takes the form of discontinuing birth attendance altogether, or obtaining employment in prenatal instruction or shift-nursing on labour and delivery wards of hospitals.

The status of midwives in Canada is unique. In 1993 only two provinces have legalized midwifery, and even in those provinces few women have ready access to qualified midwives. Largely replaced by physicians and nurses, midwives in Canada and the United States were discouraged from attending births. Childbirth was increasingly defined as a medical event to be properly supervised by medical practitioners in hospital settings. This ideology of medical control is reinforced by legislation restricting or prohibiting other forms of birth attendance and ceding monopoly powers to physicians. Many American states outlawed midwifery, and midwifery became isolated from theoretical and clinical training: "In Europe, scientific advances became incorporated into the repertoire of midwives' techniques. In the United States, on the other hand, no systematic attempts were made to upgrade the profession through training. Midwives were increasingly seen as ignorant and dirty. Childbirth passed into the medical realm, and midwifery suffered a decline that is only beginning to be reversed" (Jordan 1980, 96–7).

The development of community midwifery in Canada stems from a much wider challenge to obstetrics and gynecology. Women's reproductive health, including the ways in which birth was managed in the middle part of the twentieth century in North America, was seen as subject to medical definitions of health and excessive surgical and medical intervention. Historical accounts of midwifery in Canada show that midwives were eclipsed and nearly eradicated across Canada. Restrictive laws and ideologies surrounding birth spiralled together, establishing medicalized birth as a desirable norm, an advance that was in the interests of birthing women and in the general interest. As midwives became less prominent, the work of obstetrical and maternity-care nurses was truncated. The sphere of practice for nurses was circumscribed, with male physicians "presiding" over birth. Thus, in North America, birth attendance was increasingly defined in medical terms. Medicalization carried some benefits, such as pain relief, for patients; however, even those benefits occur within the context of a "masculinist biomedical view" (Riessman 1989, 215) ill suited to the empowerment of women. Gaskin (1988, 42) highlights the artificiality of American obstetrics: "By the 1920s, the United States had founded a truly novel custom: that of sanctioning men to make the rules and supply the knowledge for an intimately physical process that they never experienced. Lost totally to the general public was the idea that a woman could be trained to safely attend another woman in labour."

Significantly, as midwifery was being eclipsed in twentieth-century Canada, primary birth attendance was not undertaken by female physicians. Despite the role of the Ontario Medical College for Women (closed in 1906) and the subsequent establishment of Women's College Hospital, female physicians were a rarity. By 1911 only 2.7 per cent of physicians in Canada were women. This percentage fell to 1.8 per cent in 1921 (Buckley 1979, 128–9).

Medical control of birth led to a cultural transformation of birth. Attempts to connect the tradition of birth as a neighbourly and comunity-oriented event saw the formation in 1897 of the Victorian Order of Nurses (VON). Mason (1988, 107–8) depicts the VON as a movement that "threatened the doctors' prospects for hegemony over birth" more directly than other efforts to preserve traditional birth culture. The VON initiative to provide training to lay midwives generated "virtually unanimous" opposition in the medical profession. The end result was a lessening of the nursing role envisioned by VON proponents, such that members of the VON were primarily seen as fulfilling an assistant's role alongside physicians. In the traditional birth culture, women were able to assume delivery positions that were comfortable for them, in contrast to the obligatory use of the lithotomy position (in stirrups, with legs spread) used in modern obstetrical practice. "Most women tried to walk around and keep to their activities as long as possible during the first part of their labour, and squatting seems to have been common during the pushing stage" (Mason 1988, 102).

The medicalization of birth thus involved the transformation of women into receptive clients and assistants to male physicians, unable to understand or influence their own wellbeing. In her novel Surfacing, Margaret Atwood vividly described the feeling of being treated like a thing: "They shut you in a hospital, they shave the hair off you and tie your hands down, and they don't let you see, they don't want you to understand, they want you to believe it's their power, not yours. They stick needles in you so you won't hear anything, you might as well be a dead pig, your legs are up in a metal frame, they bend over you, technicians, mechanics, butchers, students clumsy or sniggering, practising on your body, they take the baby out like a pickle out of a pickle jar. After that, they fill your veins up with red plastic, I saw it running down the tube. I won't let them do that to me ever again" (cited in Treichler 1990, 118).

One woman described her experiences of childbirth in Canada in the 1950s: "I had my first baby in the mid-50s and it was impersonal and very terrifying. You went to the hospital and your husband just dropped you off. He wasn't allowed to come into the case room or the delivery room. You went into the delivery room and you were with strangers. You didn't know anybody. I think the most terrifying part for me was delivering when you were laying on your back. Your legs were strapped in stirrups, and then he strapped your hands down, so you were completely strapped down and that's how you delivered. Just before the baby was born, they put you under again and when you woke up this is when you were told if it was a boy or a girl … It was lonely, very lonely … I found all three births a terrifying experience for me" (Gerrie White, in *Midwifery and the Law* 1991).

Gerrie White compared her delivery with her first experience of seeing a live birth in 1976, when her granddaughter was born at home in Vancouver. That birth was "a very loving experience." Yet her daughter, Lee Saxell, reported that being part of the circle of friends and family at a midwife-attended birth evoked a sense of loss when she thought of how women gave birth a generation before. Lee Saxell spoke of the bridging of the two worlds of women's birth: "My mother and my aunt, her best friend, were both at the birth. When my daughter was born, they were ecstatic with the birth of the baby, but afterwards they went downstairs and they both cried their eyes out at the table. And later they told me that they realized between them, they'd delivered five babies and had never seen one born … they felt such a loss that they didn't get to experience that … the midwives were down in the kitchen with them, because they were crying … it was the joy of the birth of a grandchild, but also the loss (Lee Saxell, in *Midwifery and the Law* 1991). These experiences lend weight to the argument that births need not be controlled in ways that alienate women or their families. Today women establish birth plans that set out their expectations, such as allowing greater access for partners, husbands, or relatives, rooming-in of mothers and new-borns, and a general humanization of obstetrics, including support for midwifery services (Van Wagner 1984).

THE RE-EMERGENCE of midwifery in Canada and the United States has generated considerable resistance. In Canada, most midwives seeking legal recognition and acceptance within the health-care system have not succeeded in establishing the requirements of a distinct profession: control over their work, a self-regulating body to establish standards of care and disciplinary measures, legal protection, and specialized research and education forums. In the United States there has been some acceptance of nurse-midwifery to the extent that midwifery is established as a subspecialty of nursing. Nurse-midwifery is defined as "the independent management of care of essentially normal newborns and women, antepartally, intrapartally, postpartally, and/or gynecologically" within a system that permits collaboration and referral among other health practitioners. Moreover, nurse-midwives must meet the standards of the American College of Nurse-Midwives. In Canada, there have been attempts to place midwives within the compass of provincial nursing bodies. Nevertheless, midwives generally seek to establish midwifery as a distinct profession, with multiple routes of entry to practice. These multiple routes would include nursing training, yet would also allow for direct entry to midwifery training and certification without the requirement of nursing experience.

The midwifery movement is a valuable initiative in terms of women's health and the law. It challenges the extraordinary powers of monopoly vested in the professions, and shifts the focus in pregnancy from pathology to women's power in giving and attending birth. It also undercuts the expanded powers of the state in regulating women's health by restoring childbirth to the status of a private matter and one that is conducted, where possible, in the sphere of civil society. Midwifery advocates point to women's satisfaction with the intimate, skilled aspects of qualified midwifery care, and to several studies that testify to midwives' skill in reducing morbidity rates for mothers and infants.

There is little value, however, in asserting the benefits of contemporary community midwifery without seriously considering valid criticisms. The following sections set out the difficulties of oppositional ideologies, the emphasis on meeting the mother's wishes for delivery, the material basis of practice, the lack of formal guidelines for safe practice, and the safety of midwife-attended home births. Consideration is given to the value of legal regulation of midwifery services, and how the practice of midwifery might be altered under the auspices of the state and the professions. Recognizing midwives by allowing them a central place in maternity and infant care has been associated with reduced levels of morbidity and mortality for mothers and infants. And while these advances in safety may be most evident in developing countries (Begum, Kabir, and Mollah 1990; Nasah 1991), Canadian midwives could enhance health care here. In 1983 there were 8.5 deaths per 1,000 live births. This rate compared favourably with many other countries; for example, the Federal Republic of Germany (10.9), England and Wales (10.8), Czechoslovakia (16.9), France (9.7), Poland (20.2), Mexico (38.5), and the United States (12.6). Japan and the Netherlands had lower rates of infant mortality (6.6 and 8.3 respectively) (Statistics Canada 1986, 56).

"WE AND THEY": OPPOSITIONAL IDEOLOGIES

Many have noted the danger of oversimplifying the platforms of one's rivals. Apparent oppositions between groups or ideologies may sometimes overlap, and there is a possibility that one group claiming superiority over others may take on elements that mirror those of the discredited group.

Some midwives take an oppositional approach to medicine, hospitals, and technology, such that their resistance to institutionalized birthing may jeopardize the health of newborns and mothers. This is an ironic twist. While midwives have complained that they have been unfairly characterized as menaces to mothers and infants, it seems that some midwives are so opposed to the institution of the hospital and the staff therein that the life-saving uses of professional resources are cut off. One case in point involves the birth of an infant with respiratory difficulties after birth. The community midwife consulted with a family physician before suggesting that the child would do well at home. Unfortunately, the infant died shortly thereafter. While there is no assurance that the infant would have survived had it had hospital care, this case highlights a resistance to the use of orthodox resources and an ideology that may well overemphasize maternal-infant bonding and the superiority of home environments over hospitals. Marsden Wagner (1985, 55) alludes to a possible tendency on the part of midwives to be inflexible and dogmatic. Recently, a mother of two children editorialized against the essentialism of some advocates of natural childbirth. Barbara Wade Rose (1992) resented the ways in which some birth attendants or advocates might try to "compensate for their own disappointment" in childbirth. She added: "In such a creed, everything about home births and midwifery is 'right' and everything about hospitals and doctors is 'wrong.'" Long demonized in some western societies, some birth attendants now may be demonizing more established practitioners.

In her 1980 trial, Margaret Marsh, a spiritual healer and ex-physician, was alleged to have asked the couple, "Don't you believe in angels?" when they said they wished to transfer to hospital (*R. v. Marsh* 1980). A number of midwives I interviewed stated that midwives should transfer if the mother wishes to transfer, even if there are no tangible signs of distress.

The home birth records I studied clearly indicated that midwives are accustomed to transferring women or infants to hospital when complications arise. Beyond this, most midwives urge their clients to see a general practitioner and an obstetrical specialist if required. However, many midwives agree that a collegial spirit of working with other health professionals ought not to be translated into a subordinate position.

SERVING MOTHERS

The principle that a woman's wishes should be respected in childbirth may become problematic if the woman refuses to transfer to hospital despite the recommendations of her midwife. There are incidents where the back-up physician and the community midwife recommend hospital delivery. When the woman refuses, the midwife may support the woman's choice. The clash between respect for the client and the obligation to protect the infant (and possibly the mother) is sometimes evident in instances where a breech presentation occurs; in British Columbia two legal actions (a trial and the issuance of a warrant for the arrest of a midwife who fled the country) followed infant deaths after breech presentations in 1979 and 1980. A community midwife offered the following thoughts in 1985, just prior to two major inquests and related events in British Columbia: "If you look around, the only two deaths that have been significant [with respect to prosecution] have been breech presentations at home, and that tells quite a story in itself. I know a midwife who attempted to manage a breech at home. It was a disaster, and ended up in a transfer and a caesarean delivery. To the midwife, it wasn't a disaster; to me it was ... There are women who say that they will [deliver] anyone at home because it is a woman's right to choose where she gives birth. This is true, but on the other hand, the midwife's responsibility goes beyond the mother to the child. It is the midwife's responsibility to take both of them safely through the delivery. If someone came to the Midwives' Association adamantly wanting a breech delivery managed at home, we would refer her to a hospital."

In one instance documented by a senior midwife in Ontario, the police and paramedics were called by the midwife. The mother refused to accept the midwife's suggestion that a transfer was advisable. By calling the authorities, the midwife followed professional protocol, and her interests would have been protected if legal action was considered. Although these conflicts are rare, they underscore the dilemmas that can arise when guidelines are unavailable, or unenforceable.

There is a tendency for critics of medical intervention to interpret professional power in medicine as structured primarily to maintain "conspiracies of silence" aimed at protecting the profession's members. This instrumentalist outlook has been challenged by studies such as Bosk's (1979, 190) observations of surgical practice in the United States: "Postgraduate training of surgeons is above all things an ethical training. Subordinates are harshly disciplined when they violate the ethical standards of the discipline. They are promoted and adopted into the ranks as colleagues on the basis of their ethical fitness. It is true that the moral standards demanded and the superordinates' self-interest converge here to a high degree. Nevertheless, the point remains that normative standards of dedication, interest, and thoroughness are applied in evaluating subordinates rather than narrow technical standards."

The line drawn between "spiritual" midwifery and medical attendance obscures the hard-fought attempts of women to gain access to medical knowledge and to practise medicine. There is clearly a substantial overlap between midwifery practice and more conventional resources (laboratory work, general practice, obstetrics, and hospital resources). It would be misleading to suggest that most community midwives adhere to a strict oppositional ideology or to one that blindly follows clients' wishes. Most community midwives active in British Columbia in the 1980s have become licensed midwives and/ or registered nurses. Some are contemplating graduate studies in midwifery in England starting in 1993. The following excerpt from a letter to the *Times-Colonist* in Victoria conveys this general spirit of concern for the safety of mothers and babies and the need to combine choice in childbirth with greater interaction between midwives and other birth attendants: "As a Vancouver Island representative of the Midwives' Association of B.C., I am responding to a letter ... headed 'Home births risky' [written by the president of the provincial medical association]. The MABC is also looking forward to the establishment of a committee to investigate obstetrical care in B.C. It is indeed a tragedy whenever an unexpected death occurs during childbirth, no matter where it happens. It remains a concern for all midwives, parents and physicians that this occurs and I am sure that when it happens in the hospital, it's no less a tragedy ... The task force struck by the Ontario government in 1986 took nearly two years to complete an in-depth study and recommend the legalization of midwifery in that province. Some of the issues addressed were safety, education, qualifications and back-up. One hopes that the proposed committee for B.C. does as thorough an investigation and joins the many voices for responsible, safe and legalized midwives in this province" (Ray 1988).

SOCIAL CLASS AND MIDWIVES' CLIENTELE

Historical sources suggest that midwives have often assisted the poorer classes in many societies; the Frontier Nursing Service in rural Kentucky and the Maternity Centre Association in New York City are two examples. In recent times, however, the re-emergence of community midwifery and of nurse-midwifery in North America has been tied to the presence of a more advantaged, middle-class clientele.

Research on the class composition of midwifery clients is complicated by the different foci taken by researchers. Some concentrate on natural childbirth, others on people choosing home births or nurse-midwifery services. A study of childbirth records from thirteen hospitals in Erie County in New York state indicated that parents inclined toward natural childbirth tended to be older (on average, by two years), college-educated, white, with higher income and higher socio-economic status. These findings were reported to be consistent with earlier studies in New York City, Boston, and New Haven (Cave 1978). Citing a 1989 article on childbirth in the United States, Mitford (1992, 209) notes that women giving birth in alternative birth centres "are typically white, middle-class, over eighteen, married, college-educated, well-nourished." Other researchers noted that women with a high school or some post-secondary education had a greater need to establish personal control during labour than women with less education (Butani and Hadnett 1980, 77). Two reports on out-of-hospital births noted that women who elected home births tended to have a higher level of education than women who elected hospital births (Divorky 1981; Devitt 1979). The issue of social class has been raised with respect to birthing in England. A Community Health Council representative noted: "Criticisms are often made that organisations such as the National Childbirth Trust are very elitist and middle class in their attitudes, making it very difficult for working class women to penetrate the networks of coffee morning and afternoon teas. These criticisms are valid in that the NCT is a very powerful pressure-group pushing for natural childbirth methods which meet the needs of its predominantly healthy, well-nourished, white, middle class members. There is a danger that if the NHS is pushed into meeting their demands for non-medicalised childbirth, there may be a failure to pick up the minority of working class women at risk who do require medical intervention during labour" (Langridge, cited in CSP editors 1982, 64; but see J. Kitzinger 1990).

As set out in the previous chapter, while few mothers in the Canadian home birth sample are on social assistance, the sample is hardly uniformly advantaged. Few families enjoy above-average incomes, and to label them as "middle-class" is misleading. A second difficulty is that, given the structure of health services for parturient women in Canada, it is not possible for community midwives to remain self-employed unless they generate a sufficient income through self-employment (prenatal care, birthing attendance, post-natal visits). This is not to suggest that the equation "midwifery = middle class" is fixed. There are possibilities for extending midwifery services if midwives achieve a legitimate standing among other health care practitioners. Finally, the available literature on birth management suggests that midwives (and other birth attendants) need to tailor their care to all social classes. Some studies suggest that working-class women may have more positive attitudes toward medical intervention than middle-class women (McIntosh 1989; Nelson 1983). Clearly, for some midwives, this raises the issue of women's socialization and expectations of birth.

Another criticism involves the limitations of de facto community midwifery practice. Alan Schwartz, vice-chairman of a four-member task force studying midwifery in Ontario, has noted this concern: "[Schwartz] said [the task force] must find a way to make midwifery acceptable to a wide population that is not 'culturally attuned' to it. 'We have to ensure that it comes into the system gradually so it's not only accepted by the very small number of people today who are looking for midwives, but by the population as a whole as a real and viable alternative. It would be a great pity if you ended up with a system that ultimately serves only a very tiny percentage of the population" (Kershaw 1986, 21).

One problem with this approach is that it raises two questions: first, whether only a small number of people prefer midwifery attendance; and second, whether midwifery practice out of hospital is indeed not a "real and viable alternative." It is critically important in the discourse over midwifery to suspend any such assumptions, for there is evidence to indicate that midwifery services are desired by a good proportion of expectant mothers. Furthermore, as this study demonstrates, contemporary domiciliary practice in Canada and elsewhere need not be more dangerous than hospital-situated births managed by conventional obstetrical teams. The successful domiciliary approach would require adequate training of midwives, appropriate emergency response services, careful screening, and guidelines for practice. There is also a serious question concerning the structuring of exclusion. There is little evidence that most community midwives in British Columbia object to the possibility of working in hospital on a more independent footing. Likewise, there has been no shortage of nurse-midwives willing to participate in the demonstration projects devised in Vancouver and other parts of Canada.

MATERIAL BASIS OF PRACTICE

One aspect of midwifery practice is the material basis of practice. Community midwives are largely self-employed. While some supplement their incomes with labour coaching in hospital or other work, most are dependent on client payments. This issue is a common ground for midwives and other birth attendants. The self-interest of the medical and nursing professions in managing births is more frequently discussed than the material interests of community midwives. Subsequent research should explore the possible overlap between the ideal of midwifery and the material reality. The ideal that midwives should attend even high-risk births may dovetail with some midwives' interest in generating a sufficient income. Dr. Sidney Sharzer, the chief of the obstetrics and gynecology department in a Los Angeles hospital, has been quoted on the issue of monetary self-interest and what in his view appears to be a hypercritical approach by some midwives toward hospital-based maternity care. "Sharzer thinks midwives are out to make a buck like anyone else. And, he says, they have overestimated the demand for 'natural' births. Since the public demand for alternative birthing is low, 'they've got to emphasize negative things that go on in a hospital to draw business.' Hospitals, too, he says, 'are concerned with personalizing the birth experience'" (Mittelbach 1986, 10).

Once again, the possibility of midwives' making a living from the community appears to have run its course for most community midwives of a decade ago in British Columbia. Community midwifery, with its long hours, legal uncertainties, and low pay, seems to be best suited to more formal integration in the health-care system, notwithstanding concerns about "watered-down" midwifery care because of needless regulation by the other health professions.

FORMAL STRUCTURE, IDIOSYNCRATIC PRACTICE?

Another important issue is the need to establish standards of practice while granting discretion to practising midwives. Unlike nurse-midwives, obstetrical nurses, and physicians, the community midwife movement in British Columbia has not yet generated a clear and enforceable set of guidelines for practice. To carry on in the absence of formal standards of practice, provision for peer review, and a range of penalties creates a risk that practice will become idiosyncratic and unsafe. The 1984 coroner's inquest in Toronto followed the delivery of an infant on an island. The distance from hospital and the speed of transportation may be factors to be considered in deciding whether or not to attend a home delivery; so may be the need to have more than one midwife present at a birth in the event that complications arise for the mother and infant.

In 1986 a community midwife with experience in only a few primary care deliveries attended a mother in labour on an island in British Columbia. In retrospect, there might have been concerns about a relatively junior midwife's managing a birth in a locale where emergency assistance was limited. Nevertheless, the birth proceeded without complications, and no formal complaint was made to the Midwives Association of British Columbia. It is arguable that the midwife could have refused to attend, citing the delay in transporting from an island to hospital, the need for a more experienced midwife, and the limited number of prenatal visits by the attending midwife. As it happened, the birth was uneventful; however, this case dramatized the tension between private agreements between midwives and clients and the public concern over safe practice. Midwives may answer that they are cautious in agreeing to attend clients who do not live near them. One community midwife spoke about her practice in the mid-1980s:

I have been on Vancouver Island, a few Gulf Islands, and up to the northern interior of B.C. It is relatively common for the midwives practising in Vancouver, because quite often they will get a call from people out of town where there are no facilities, no practising midwives in their area, and the hospital routine is so awful. These people want alternative birthing, and it just isn't available to them in their community hospitals ... Things are improving, but there is still a long way to go. In the little, outlying hospital so much depends on who the physician is ... Sometimes clients come down to see me. What I did with my people was to get a copy of their prenatal records from their doctors who knew they were going to have a home birth ... I would go about a week early, depending on their history. All the clients I have had from out of town were having their second or third baby, and quite often I had already been involved with the delivery of the first, so I know the people. They have had a really straightforward history, without any complicating factors.

Certainly the gap between the formal structure of midwives' associations and the specific practices of members has not been satisfactorily addressed. Doctors and nurses have been critical of midwives' delays in transferring women from home to hospital if, for example, bradycardia (a drop in the fetal heart rate) is manifested during labour. Concerns have also been voiced about misjudgments by midwives managing home births. A Vancouver physician who is openly supportive of midwifery expressed some misgivings about certain midwifery practices during his testimony in the 1986 Sullivan-LeMay trial in Vancouver. The doctor "said he can understand the reasons people choose for home births, such as feeling more comfortable in a familiar setting to a distrust of hospitals, but he 'would have some scruples' about attending home deliveries himself. 'There are some children who have not survived which I feel might have if they'd been delivered in hospital'" (Banks 1986, B6).

Another aspect of midwifery practice that has attracted some criticism is variation in record-keeping. Community midwives in Canada have not produced a systematic study of their practices and birth outcomes. This reflects in large measure the time devoted to prenatal assessments and consultations, labour and delivery, and postnatal care and visits. The situation is not helped, however, by uneven patterns of documentation in the 1970s in British Columbia. Some births receive only cursory documentation; many others are accompanied by precise, detailed notations of prenatal and postnatal care and labour and delivery processes. A related problem is that midwives have not established a collation of attempted home births through a central agency, and it is very difficult to discern patterns of practice, let alone analyse the central issue of maternal and infant health.

These difficulties have been compounded by the apparent reluctance of some midwives to establish a standardized set of charts for practice. Standardization would allow comparisons of such variables as time of the stages of labour and the social class and occupation of the mother (and partner, where applicable). The latter would be a useful addition to birth records, given the association between socio-economic status and infant mortality, as mentioned earlier. On a broader scale, the absence of standardized collection procedures hinders research and development possibilities for community midwives. It is virtually impossible to monitor transfer rates to hospitals, birth weights of newborns, types of deliveries, and a host of other variables unless there is a comprehensive data base. The absence of standardization reduces the possibility of midwives' learning from each other's practices, and lessens the kinds of statistical contributions they could make to other midwifery associations and publications. Flint (1986, 134–40) offers a thoughtful discussion on the merits of keeping a thorough "booking history" for clients. Paine (1991) favours more accurate information on midwives' work. She believes that without such information midwives' contributions may be ignored. Midwifery practice and research are thus integral parts of promoting midwives' status: "This knowledge about practice is the beginning of the midwife's power base of information. She will have regained the essential information needed to elevate her professional status" (Paine 1991, 202).

Clearly, there is a contradiction between the need for comprehensive documentation of birth attendance and outcomes, and the very limited infrastructure of research resources available to the community midwives and to nurse-midwives. We can hardly expect midwives to produce reliable statistics when they are limited by their illegal or alegal status, and do not have direct access to hospital, regional, or provincial data bases. If structure serves to discourage scientific analyses of midwifery practice, however, it is not completely prohibitive. Some Canadian midwives have produced statistics on their practices. Moreover, there is considerable interest on the part of midwives in contributing to research on midwifery practice, as evidenced by the strong support provided for this present study and other studies of Canadian midwives. It is important to note that research attributed to midwives tends to be regarded (by midwives) as less important than research attributed to physicians (Hicks 1992). It is encouraging to learn, however, that as part of the continuing education of graduates of the British Columbia School of Midwifery a session was convened to discuss the principles of research and writing, including the development of standardized birth records that would facilitate computer analysis. Research and writing skills have also been emphasized by the architects of a master's degree in midwifery practice at Queen Charlotte's hospital and Thames Valley University in London.

HOSPITALS AND
THE EXPANDED ROLE
OF NURSE-MIDWIVES

Another possibility is that the role of obstetrical nurses might be expanded. The nurses could help to meet the public demand for hospital-based midwifery. The counter-argument is that the nurses might be co-opted into a dependent role, even if their sphere of practice was expanded. This argument may be too dismissive. Midwifery attendance could be brought within the ambit of provincial nursing legislation such that nurses would be more self-directing in managing births. In fact, the legislation now being developed in Ontario relies heavily on input from nurse-midwives for its implementation. It is also noteworthy that the Midwives' Program in place in the Grace Hospital in Vancouver has been designated as a "functional program" in the hospital budget. This means that the hospital board has endorsed the program as an integral part of labour and delivery services, and the program will be evaluated or reviewed by the board. Moreover, Doctors' Hospital in Toronto has presented a brief to a legislative task force in Ontario proposing the development of clinical training for midwives in conjunction with the medical and nursing faculties at the University of Toronto (*Whig-Standard* 1986).

It is also possible that hospital services could be altered to become more client-oriented, more humanizing, and less oriented toward interventions. The hospital or an adjacent birthing centre could meet some of the demands for reformed childbirth practices, and it offers rapid access to emergency measures in the event of cord prolapses, hemorrhage, fetal decelerations, and other complications of childbirth. As some have suggested, however, it is questionable whether hospital staff are making drastic reductions in interventions. Further, birthing rooms are not as yet proliferating in hospitals. Nevertheless, if midwives are given hospital privileges or are allowed to work on a salaried basis, then the home birth option may become less frequent.

A related point is that legalized midwifery, whether practised by nurse-midwives or direct-entry midwives (who would not require a separate degree or diploma in nursing), might become as bureaucratic and restrictive as other components of Canadian health care. This possibility rekindles earlier commentary in this chapter: what is lost when human services become more formal and health practices become increasingly controlled by the professions? A danger is that as community midwifery becomes subject to peer review (or outside review), midwives are more likely to be suspended or otherwise disciplined than if they practised independently. It is likely that midwives' current autonomy will be reduced if midwifery is legally recognized. Some will suggest that legalization of midwifery will correct for idiosyncratic and risky practices, but others fear that the special relationship of community midwife and client will be compromised as midwives become state-controlled. Clients may likewise be precluded from obtaining midwifery services if they are deemed to be at high risk. Once again the state or the professions will emerge as mediators of community decisions, particularly if health services become more centralized and bureaucratic.

Criticisms of midwifery practice need to be kept in context. First, it is misleading to speak of midwives as a totality, for practices and philosophies vary markedly among midwives. For example, some will accept high-risk clients, while others will not. Second, some of these criticisms highlight isolated concerns that may arise but are not indicative of the usual processes of midwife-client interaction. Nevertheless, for the reasons outlined above, there is a danger in merely advocating community midwifery as a good. Risks may be taken on the grounds of spiritual idealism; record-keeping may be unsystematic and difficult to assess in the aggregate; and the emphasis on empowering the woman in labour may obscure wider concerns such as the class or ethnic composition of clients served by community midwives in British Columbia and elsewhere. Midwives counter that they would prefer to serve a broader socio-economic range of clients, but since midwifery is outlawed and must generate private income (outside the provincial medical billing plans) it will attract clients who can afford to pay for private midwifery services. A key point here is that midwives have become more self-critical of their work, and have stepped up research activities and clinical skills on many fronts.

Self-regulation contributes to the freedom of practising midwives and their distance from controlling bureaucracies. Self-regulation can become problematic when one considers the established regulation of other professions involved in childbirth, along with the general trend toward rational bureaucratic systems in law and health care. The classic formulation of legal-rational domination was set out by Max Weber. In *Economy and Society,* bureaucratic rationality is cast as an impartial system of rules. Ideally, this system of rules and formal procedures is not controlled by bureaucrats for their own interests. The contemporary critique of technologically based childbirth management indicates, however, that the client and the community can be engulfed as their power is replaced by professional control over childbirth.

MAKING A DIFFERENCE:
WOMEN'S PREFERENCES IN
BIRTH

Just a note to thank you for your support, caring and direction during the birth of our baby. Without you I don't know if we would have been able to stick to our birth plan of almost no medications, and no episiotomy. You made the team work.

I just want to write to you to once again say "thank you" so much for all your help during my labour on Sunday. I honestly cannot thank you enough. I have never ever been in more pain in my life. My first two deliveries were easy compared to the intensity of Sunday's experience. Without your knowledge and guidance and total devotion to me during that time, I think I would have lost my mind. I can't imagine a more supportive person than you. You go so far beyond the call of duty. I just thank God that you were on shift when I was in labour (Notes to midwife Carol Hird; see Burtch 1992).

Much of the medical discourse on childbirth centres on the importance of safety in childbirth. Culturally speaking, the death of an infant at term or a serious injury to a newborn child can be viewed as a major loss – an emotional loss for the parents and, given the possibility of litigation, a loss of legitimacy for the hospital and attendants. In over a thousand home birth records from Ontario, British Columbia, and Saskatchewan, most clients placed less emphasis on morbidity or death in birth, concentrating on preparation for childbirth. Preparations for birth – diet, exercise, prenatal examination, physician back-up, and hospital access – were often emphasized (Burtch 1988). Thus, while midwives and their clients are likely to discuss the prospect of infant loss, this is not the overriding feature of interactions with their midwives. The nature of modern obstetrics and legal practice has nevertheless been recast, transforming loss in childbirth as a problematic event that may well result in civil litigation against caregivers. In the United States, midwives are increasingly being required to carry malpractice insurance. In Canada, the Task Force on the Implementation of Midwifery in Ontario (1987) recommended that midwives carry such insurance.

Midwives tend to be flexible in their practices. Most have experience in assisting women in hospital by acting as labour coaches. In addition, for community midwives in Canada, home birth is a source of income and more autonomous experience in labour and birth attendance. What is striking about their work and their records is the willingness of midwives to respect their clients' wishes. In many cases, there is a quality of reassurance for women who, having delivered a baby in hospital, are now seeking to give birth at home. Similarly, midwives can reassure clients who wish to give birth at hospital, having already had a home birth. The following extract is taken from a letter written in 1989 to a community midwife: "Since our conversation last week I've felt so much better. I still feel that this time we should birth in hospital. It was real interesting to know that I could have chosen a homebirth too & that you would have been available, willing etc, & yet deep down I felt better about hospital! ... I want to say 'thank you' for taking the time to listen, for understanding & for your thoughtful words of advice. We have such wonderful memories of you from past births, I'm sure I'll think of you in labour!"

Women's preferences in childbirth have not been a central focus of scholarly work on maternity and infant care. However, there has been a growing critical literature that documents women's dissatisfaction with many features of modern obstetrics. This work includes interviews with women following birth, and general critiques of the medicalization of childbirth (Oakley 1984; Rothman 1984; Ginzberg, 1989; Hird and Burtch 1991; Mitford 1992). The socialization of physicians has also been criticized for its emphasis on unnecessary intervention and fragmented care for women.

The literature has often linked historical practices with modern obstetrical structures and practices. Martin refers to the power of the metaphor of the body as machine in seventeenth- and eighteenth-century French medical research and practice. LaMettrie's influential treatise, "Man, the Machine," made an analogy between human bodies (as functioning or malfunctioning machines) and the appeal of medical intervention, using such "mechanical devices" as the forceps. Reliance on these medical devices "played a great part in the replacement of female midwives' hands by male hands using tools" (Martin 1987, 140–3). Concerns have been raised about the costs of using high technology in health care. This technology absorbs millions of dollars but serves only a small fraction of the population (see Jordan 1987). Some favour greater autonomy for midwives in reducing unnecessary interventions such as caesarean sections and routine epidurals (Wagner 1990).

Significantly, even as the medical and nursing disciplines established medical control over various stages of pregnancy and childbirth, there have been objections to the treatment of women in maternity wards. Kitzinger, reviewing letters and other sources concerning women giving birth in England, likens some of their feelings to those associated with women who have been raped or otherwise violated (Kitzinger 1990). Stanko (1990: 97) uses the concept of "little rapes" to denote the everyday indignities, humiliations, and threats that affect many women. We can draw a parallel between women's feeling restricted in their movements and their sense of security, and the discomfort of some women in current birth settings and practices. This feeling of being discounted or devalued is clearly tied to other reports of how "femaleness" may be disregarded or insulted in many cultures (Renzetti and Curran 1989). The midwifery movement, recognizing an obstetrical field that may operate at the expense of women, seeks to empower women in birthing choices.

Empowerment can take many forms. These range from collective action, such as lobbying for legal recognition of autonomous midwifery, to individual acts against medicalization. Martin recognizes patterns of resistance by expectant women to medicalized childbirth. She notes the establishment of childbirth activist groups that offer guides to "self-defence in the hospital." Mothers may also deliberately delay their trip to hospital as a strategy of reducing the likelihood of intervention by hospital staff (if the labour does not progress according to their expectations). Martin indicates that once in the hospital, some women unstrap fetal monitors or take extended walks or showers – activities that give them greater privacy and freedom of movement during labour. For Martin, such tactics stand as methods of resistance by women to an interfering, interventionistic approach to managing births. She concludes that the decision to give birth at home – a decision that is generally denounced by medical and nursing associations in Canada and elsewhere – may be "the most effective tactic" in women's reclaiming birth (Martin 1987, 140–3).

Against the power of the machine-metaphor of birth, women's agency in leaving, delaying, concealing, and opting out of conventional birth care is celebrated. This is not to reduce these and other actions to mere resistance: much of the critical literature recognizes women's power in childbirth as well as the importance of ritual celebrations of women's integrity. One example of this is midwifery practice that allows women greater freedom of choice in delivery positions. The lithotomy position has become conventional in obstetrics; but many women in Canada use other positions in home births. This finding matches evidence that delivery positions other than a supine position have been used in many cultures (Hedstrom and Newton 1986, 182–3). A growing body of scientific literature supports a less interventionistic approach. For example, Klein and his associates (1983, 1993) have explored the use of episiotomy by North American physicians. They recommend that the liberal or routine practice of episiotomy be discontinued. Episiotomy

should only be utilized for specific fetal indications such as evidence that birth must be expedited for reasons of fetal distress or of clear maternal indications, such as the woman's inability to give birth without an instrumental intervention. It should be kept in mind that this recommendation can only be implemented in a context in which the birth attendant is trained for, and is skilled in, the protection of the perineum from severe trauma. In fact, even the use of forceps and vacuum extractions are not absolute indications for utilizing episiotomy. The acquisition of skills in the use of vacuum extraction and forceps is also recommended (Klein et al., 1993).

Reviewing the work of Sheila Kitzinger, two researchers contrast the "splendid ritual" of technocratic births with modern attempts to restore a new sense of "identity and respect" for birthing women. The "splendid ritual" in many hospitals "affects all women no matter what their economic status ... Through its procedures, women are removed not only from their personal identities but from the actual birth and are drawn into medical rites as zealously guarded as any ceremony in the old cultures. Step by step, the woman is divested of all that is familiar in a bionic environment where she is totally dependent on strangers who themselves rely on machines for information. Inherent to this new ritual is the belief that the machines are faultless, truthful, and indispensable in the delivery of a healthy baby" (see Edwards and Waldorf 1984, 140).

PROFESSIONAL SUPPORT AND RESISTANCE

It is commonplace to pit an emerging group against more established health professions. One of the difficulties with this tactic is that there are differences of opinion *within* these health professions. Midwives differ over some aspects of practice, qualifications, and legal status (Benoit 1991). For years, community midwives have shared information about physicians who are supportive of midwifery practices. Beyond this, official position statements on the midwifery question have been formulated by medical and nursing associations. In some cases there is fairly strong support for implementing midwifery services. Even so, most medical and nursing associations express concern over the home birth option. A statement on midwifery approved by the Society of Obstetricians and Gynecologists of Canada (1986) noted that there was "a large amount of work to do" before midwifery could be established in Canada. Nevertheless, the SOGC recognized that "certified, licensed midwives play a major role in provision of services to pregnant women in most western countries." The statement referred to "a widely recognized exodus" of physicians – both general practitioners and specialists in obstetrics and gynecology – from obstetrical care in Canada. The society expressed concern over proper standards of training and practice for midwives in Canda. The SOGC is also on record as disapproving of home births. Birth attendance, other than that in accredited institutions such as hospitals or birthing centres, should be discouraged: "The issue of home births is often confused with the introduction of midwifery. The Society of Obstetricians and Gynecologists of Canada believes that these are two (2) entirely different issues. Our Society wishes to re-emphasize its policy that *"Ideally all deliveries should occur in an accredited hospital maternal unit. We strongly disapprove of home births as not being in the best interest of either mothers or infants. Any free standing childbirth centre should have a physical and organizational attachment to an existing accredited maternity centre.* Introduction of nurse midwifery or midwifery does not alter this policy" (SOGC 1986, 4 [emphasis in original]).

Professional views on midwifery appear to be divided. The hegemonic view of birth as a medical event, requiring professional care within established guidelines, does not require that midwifery should be eradicated. Some observers point to differences of opinion among physicians over the value of midwifery. An obstetrician recalled the results of one survey of doctors in British Columbia: "It is my feeling, from talking to a lot of family physicians across the province, that you are probably looking at a 50–50 balance. Fifty per cent would be in support of some kind of midwifery ... either working with them in the office, or in the hospital, or in a referral pattern. Another 50 per cent would be either uneasy, or strictly opposed ... When I was involved in the Executive of the B.C. Medical Association section of Obstetricians and Gynaecologists, I at some stage sent out questionnaires to the obstetricians and gynaecologists in this province who were practising obstetrics. At that time, 75 per cent were in support of some type of midwifery in this province" (Bernd Wittmann, interview transcript from *Midwifery and the Law* 1991).

A statement in the *Canadian Medical Association Journal* provided little support for autonomous midwifery services in Canada. The statement followed a reformist line, suggesting that high-quality obstetrical care could be provided by existing personnel. Specifically, nurses could assume greater responsibility in obstetrical care, but under the direction of physicians (Baker 1990, 24).

The Registered Nurses' Association of British Columbia has also considered the possibility of implementing midwifery as an established health profession. In its 1978 *Position Statement on Midwifery*, the RNABC supported nurse-midwifery as an extension of nursing practice. The statement also indicated that qualified nurse-midwives could participate in care during pregnancy, labour, and delivery (and presumably in the post-partum period). The statement endorsed the sentiment of the Western Nurse Midwives Association that the health care system in Canada is not able to support home births: specifically, it cannot provide "back-up support services for emergencies." It is especially significant that the RNABC board of directors continues to envision only nurse-midwifery as a health profession. In its 1987 statement, the RNABC acknowledged the work of "non-nurse midwives," but stopped short of endorsing them as bona fide midwives: "[RNABC] is not convinced that the non-nurse midwife is a viable concept in the British Columbia health care system at this time. RNABC does not therefore support the concept of midwifery as an autonomous and self-regulating health discipline ... RNABC is strongly opposed to the practice of midwifery by unqualified and unregulated persons who have neither the necessary education nor [the] legal authority to practice in the midwife role" (RNABC 1987, 22).

This "middle position" (Cutshall 1987) on midwifery has not been set in stone. Although the RNABC board has twice established a position more conservative than that recommended by two special committees that were struck to consider issues in midwifery, it is also on record as wishing to promote further discussion among its membership. As it stands, however, the RNABC's official position lends no support to autonomous midwifery practice, including out-of-hospital deliveries or deliveries by community midwives. Interestingly, in the 1987 position statement, the community midwife is recast as "non-nurse midwife," or a "lay midwife."

The status of midwives hinges in part on the perceived need for professional birth attendants. In Ontario and Quebec, with the highest proportion of obstetricians to population, less than one-half of all births are attended by family physicians (Anderson 1986, 12). As family physicians become less prominent in labour and delivery, the case for midwifery services rests on the need for specialized care (for uncomplicated labours and deliveries), and especially on the need for rapport and continuity of care between birth attendants and pregnant women. It is clear that most community midwives – active or "retired" – are not eager to have the implementation of midwifery controlled by nursing associations. The midwifery movement now stresses cooperation among various health professions, but in such a way that the integrity of autonomous midwifery practice is preserved. For example, in its presentation to the Health Professions Council of British Columbia, the Midwives Association of British Columbia (MABC) challenged the policy of the RNABC to try to "envelop" midwifery as a part of nursing. The MABC (1993, 2) drew a clear distinction between nursing and midwifery: "Nurses do not practice midwifery – they perform nursing functions that may overlap with midwifery practice." Anderson (1986, 12) reports that midwives'

associations in British Columbia, Ontario, and Quebec favour legislation that ensures the autonomy of midwives. Legalization that would
place midwives in a dependent position below physicians or nurses
has consistently been resisted. Flint (1986) draws an analogy to other
professions, such as dentistry and law, in which formal education is
centred on these disciplines, without "sidelines." In one hypothetical
example – if, before becoming a lawyer, one would have to be trained
as a police officer – she suggests: "It's very useful for you to be a
policeman first – you learn about the criminal mind, you learn a lot
of basics of the law, you learn about court procedure, you learn how
law affects ordinary people." Flint's point is that while there may be
advantages to adjunctive studies, midwifery stands as a discipline in
its own right. Blurring the line between midwifery and nursing might
be harmful in developing optimal care for mothers and newborns.

Flint (1986) argues for a rethinking of how midwives are trained,
noting that while direct entry to midwifery practice is possible in the
United Kingdom, most midwives have been trained as nurses first.
Nursing training would not be a prerequisite for midwifery education.

In Canada, many midwives see the argument for nurse-midwifery
as compromising the special relationship between client and midwife.
Placing midwives under the supervision of physicians and within the
compass of nursing would artificially restrict midwives' skills. It would
also undermine continuity of care for expectant mothers, as midwifery
would be assimilated within the conventional structures of the obstetrical team within hospitals. Baker (1990, 24–5) makes a strong argument against a compromised status for midwives. Midwives would
be more restricted if they were regulated by provincial colleges of
nursing than if they were a self-regulating profession. Without cooperation between physicians and midwives, "legalization and regulation would not be meaningful" (Baker 1990, 24).

MIDWIFERY INITIATIVES AND CONFLICTS

The end of law is not to abolish or restrain, but to preserve and enlarge
freedom. For in all states of created beings, capable of laws, where there is
no law there is no freedom. For liberty is to be free from restraint and
violence from others; which cannot be where there is no law; and is not, as
we are told, a liberty for every man to do what he lists (John Locke, cited
in Stein and Shand 1974, 184).

The equation of law with liberty has often been challenged, and
certainly in this postmodern era. Throughout the review of the history and cultural variations of midwifery, the contradictory nature of

state regulation is crucial to an understanding of midwifery practice in Canada and elsewhere. These contradictions include the sense that western law is accepted in large measure because it provides a needed framework of rules and sanctions (Cotterrell 1984, 161–2). Yet this legal framework can serve to constrain initiatives that might equally receive public support, such as alternatives to established health services. The illegal status of many practising midwives in Canada does not clearly reflect a widespread consensus *against* community midwives and *for* physicians and obstetrical nurses. It is likely that public opinion strongly favours standards of care and certification of midwives, but there is no clear evidence that the midwifery conflict began with grave misgivings on the part of the populace. Indeed, folkways seem to protect the importance of local midwives. The point is that the redefinition of midwifery as a menace or, by way of faint praise, as a stepping-stone to obstetrical science, was generated within the predominantly male preserve of medicine and science, with considerable support from the nursing profession. While professing their monopolies to be in the general interest, these professions have failed to demonstrate that midwifery services are inherently inferior to their services, are more expensive, or are not preferred by a good number of expectant mothers. And there is ample evidence in support of the competency and affordability of certain midwifery services. A failing on the part of the midwives is that because of their uneven documentation of their own practices they have not always been able to demonstrate their competency or even the changes in their practices over time. Gaskin and Gaskin (1979, 935–42) noted that some practising midwives have maintained a careful record of out-of-hospital births they attend.

Two distinct forms of midwifery have appeared in British Columbia, Ontario, and other provinces in recent years. Nurse-midwifery as a practice separate from physicians' decisions has been aligned with projects based in hospitals. To date there has been little success in establishing out-of-hospital birthing centres in Canada, although there are models available in other countries and some nurse-midwives have sought funding to establish such centres. In contrast, community midwifery is an initiative rooted in spiritual aspects of birth and the home as a preferred site for birthing. Lacking legal status, these midwives have had greater scope of practice than professional nurse-midwives; however, unlike their professional counterparts, they have been liable to prosecution for alleged breaches of criminal and quasi-criminal law.

A conflict, then, has occurred with state officials administering provincial and federal laws. This conflict is intermittent in the sense that midwives are usually prosecuted only if there is an infant or maternal death or an injury associated with a home birth. Further-more, such injuries or deaths are often processed through coroners' inquiries and seldom through the criminal courts. State authorities in Canada have not been very proactive in prosecuting midwives for the quasi-criminal offence of practising medicine without a license. These intermittent actions should not obscure the importance of this struggle for control. The dominant approach has been to view state regulation of midwives as legitimate. Following the original convic-tion of Mary Sullivan and Gloria LeMay for criminal negligence causing death, a newspaper editorial advocated the need for state control to ensure standards of competence and safety. The journalist concluded that "a situation in which unlicensed midwives operate in a *sub rosa* atmosphere is extremely unhealthy" (Anonymous 1986a).

This pressure to regulate midwifery may reflect the limited informal sanctions brought against community midwives through existing associations. The regulations and principles currently being developed by local midwives may need to be situated within the state's ambit if the sanctions they recommend are to be implemented. These sanctions could include fines, suspensions from practice, and expulsion from the association. The larger theoretical question is whether legalization of midwifery is in fact a successful challenge to medical dominance. DeVries (1985, 129–30, 140) contends that licensed midwives are at greater risk of licence revocation or suspen-sion. Furthermore, the state's sanctioning of midwifery practice can reinforce and formalize the dominance of physicians over licensed midwives. Jessica Mitford (1992, 239–40) chronicled the defeat of a midwifery bill in California in early 1992. Despite a coalition of nurses, midwives, and supporters, the California Medical Association mounted a successful lobby against the bill.

At the same time that there is a clear statist tendency in Canada regarding freedom in childbirth, there are anomalies in the contain-ment of midwifery. Coroners' inquests in Ontario have resulted in recommendations that midwifery be granted legal standing, and none of the inquests into infant deaths after midwife-attended home births was followed by criminal prosecution of the midwives.

The tendency to prize state control over community control of birth may be offset by a central contradiction in health care in western nation-states. The fiscal crisis in these nations has prompted cutbacks in state expenditures in health and social welfare. The cap on the Canada Assistance Plan, known as the "cap on CAP," foreshadows greater efforts to reduce state expenditures and government indebt-edness. Clearly, the growth of technological approaches to illness and to childbirth pose substantial costs to the state. One method of reducing these costs is to discourage routine use of drugs and surgical interventions, and to promote the use of less expensive paramedical workers as health practitioners (Hanft and Eichenholz 1980, 151).

SELF-DETERMINATION IN REPRODUCTION AND WORK

The basic freedom of the world is woman's freedom. A free race cannot be born of slave mothers. A woman enchained cannot choose but give a measure of that bondage to her sons and daughters. No woman can call herself free who does not own and control her body. No woman can call herself free until she can choose consciously whether she will or will not be a mother (Sanger, quoted in Rossi 1976, 533).

Margaret Sanger's observations in *Woman and the New Race* (1935) are pertinent to an understanding of midwifery initiatives today. The theme of interference with women's freedom to determine the nature of the birthing experience was consistently articulated by community midwives' clients when they stated their reasons for choosing home birth. The issue of unnecessary interference with midwifery practice recurred in interviews with practising midwives, in their presentations to government associations and tribunals, and in midwifery journals and newsletters.

These conflicts between practitioners, clients, and the state should not be restricted to the contemporary conflict. As noted earlier, there has been a centuries-long conflict between physicians, nurses, and lay midwives in Europe, a conflict that encompassed the prosecution of midwives and healers for witchcraft and that was marked by the superior position of the medical profession in managing deliveries in many countries. These historical conflicts continue in contemporary debates over the place of midwifery. The British Columbia College of Physicians and Surgeons has strongly discouraged its members from professional contacts with midwives practising outside of obstetrical nursing. The Registered Nurses' Association of British Columbia, the Ontario Nurses' Association, and the Alberta College of Physicians and Surgeons have declared that their members ought not to participate in planned out-of-hospital births.

The discourse of midwifery tends to be predictable. Proponents of various forms of midwifery provide various sets of statistics (usually from places other than Canada) favourable to midwifery. Nurses and physicians either object to midwifery initiatives or allow for midwifery only if it is hospital-based and medically supervised. A recent article on midwifery in British Columbia shows how community midwifery is misrepresented by its critics. The possibility of multiple routes of entry to autonomous midwifery training is bypassed, and reappears, condesendingly, as "lay" midwifery. Consumers become invisible and voiceless; the importance of midwives' earning less than physicians is reinforced; and the continuity of care and intimacy of midwifery (key aspects of the work of many midwives in home, clinic, or hospital settings) are cast into doubt. The role of these legitimate sources of media authority is reinforced, as the midwifery initiative seemingly requires the imprimatur of physicians, nurses, and government authorities:

[A Health Ministry representative] said the ministry plans to consult with the Registered Nurses Association of B.C. and possibly explore additional midwifery pilot projects such as the one currently in place at Grace Hosptial in Vancouver. But Dr. Mary Donlevy, B.C. branch president of the Federation of Medical Women of Canada, questioned whether the government will actually save money by using nurses as midwives … She also questioned whether midwives would be involved with child delivery from pre-natal through to post-partum care. Sue Rothwell, president of the Registered Nurses Association of B.C., said Dunlevy is probably correct in saying that doctors can perform deliveries cheaper than nurses. But she emphasized that she had no facts to back up her position. But Rothwell praised the move toward designating trained nurses as midwives rather than using lay midwives. "There may be a place for lay midwives but we don't know yet" (Griffin 1988, C2).

The original research discussed in chapter four contributes to this discourse, for it appears that the idealized promotion of midwifery and its denunciation are inadequate for an understanding of its complex relations with clients, other professions, and the state. This research accents the discrepancy between what midwifery is in Canada, its more autonomous status in many other countries, and the form it might take in Canada. Internationally, midwifery has been well established as an integral part of maternity and infant care. In Canada, midwifery is only now being considered as an entity distinct from medicine and nursing.

The structuring of the conflicts between midwives (and midwifery proponents) and rival professions has occurred primarily through legal measures. These measures include the redefinition of lay midwifery as an offence under various Medical Acts. Various legal cases were mounted to prosecute these "irregular" practitioners, thereby protecting the income and status of physicians and surgeons. The Criminal Code has also been activated against Canadian midwives since 1983. The conflict, originally structured in terms of the conserving power of law, tended to portray midwifery as unsafe, as an aberration in an evolving health network. In this respect legal measures have seemed part of a rational political order that is alleged to protect a general public interest (Burtch 1992). It is crucial to weigh abstract jurisprudential principles against the effect of law on social relations. In other words, how are abstract principles of jurisprudence actually translated into the "living law?" (Burtch 1992, 69). It is also important to note counter-definitions of how birth is managed; how, for instance, certified nurse-midwives (CNMS) and independent midwives alike have received considerable support from authorities in reproductive care (Boston Women's Health Collective 1992, 409–12).

It is argued here that the state has largely served to consolidate the power of the medical and nursing professions over childbirth. Indeed, the redefinition of birth and death (from natural events to processes where injuries or deaths can generate civil, quasi-criminal, or criminal charges) carries profound implications for the limits of social change with respect to midwifery. As Foucault (1977) noted of the disciplinary society, discourse and surveillance serve to produce "docile bodies." Obedience becomes normal, disobedience becomes suspect and may be dealt with punitively. The community of women thus is mediated through much larger structures of power and knowledge as these events become cast as medical events. At the same time, knowledge is fluid not fixed. New ideas can emerge to challenge the typecasting of power and deference.

An alternative way of perceiving birth was evident in many of the birth documents. Clients tended to weigh the risks of home birth against its benefits, and to anticipate congenital abnormalities that would not be linked to the midwives' care. The following excerpt from a birth record outlines one woman's feelings about preventable and unpreventable difficulties in a home birth situation: "Hemorrhage – feel it can be dealt with appropriately by midwife and doctor – it is a slight risk. Baby has trouble breathing – also feel you are prepared for this. Baby might be grossly deformed and die as a result of lack of support systems at home. We feel this would be a natural consequence and would not regret home delivery."

PROMOTING MIDWIFERY, PROSECUTING MIDWIVES

Understanding midwifery in its Canadian context requires a sense of its complexities, not just with respect to the management of births but with respect to its relationship to obstetrical science and the state.

Midwifery in Canada is an anomaly. Despite the legal presence of midwifery in other countries and the proven competence of trained midwives, midwifery is either illegal or of uncertain legal status in all provinces of Canada (except for Ontario and Alberta). Two puzzles – the resistance to independent midwifery practice, and recent initiatives to restore midwifery – have been addressed through the contradictions of the state. These contradictions include the promotion of safe maternity and infant care (and the lag in legal recognition of midwifery) and the promotion of women's choices in reproduction and work (and the contradictory promotion of mandatory hospitalization for birth and restrictions on midwifery as an occupation). The contradictions are fused in the promotion of midwifery worldwide through such agencies as the World Health Organization and health departments or ministries in many nations, and the intermittent prosecution of practising community midwives in Canada.

These contradictions are evident in media portrayals of midwifery. On the one hand, newsmaking tends to focus on the most dramatic aspects of midwifery and birth, especially when there is an infant death associated with an attempted home birth. The continual focus on public safety and the need for greater regulation of midwives thus presents midwifery as a social problem, an unhappy situation that merits greater discipline and accountability. On the other hand, the media does provide a forum for alternatives images of birth. Patricia Graham (1987, 37), then an editorial writer for the *Vancouver Province*, offered a detailed account of her reasons for giving birth at home: "Some might say that we were lucky, but I don't believe that. I say we were responsible. I thnk that if everyone who wanted a home birth followed the precautions we took there would be little chance of anything going wrong. I think we must all be cautious about judging home births on the basis of the unfortunate stories that make the news, for those are the ones where something has gone dreadfully and needlessly wrong. And obviously the province should act quickly to educate, license and regulate midwives."

To promote midwifery, one must have access to comparative analyses of midwifery practice in hospital and other settings. Such access requires the cooperation of practising midwives in documenting their work and charting the progress of labour and delivery. Standardized forms would be useful for comparisons within British Columbia, and might be extended to other provinces and to jurisdictions outside Canada. My experience has been that community midwives will share their documents, but few have time for or interest in compiling a systematic, statistical evaluation of their work. In contrast, there have been many published accounts of nurse-midwife projects, and these could be encouraged for purposes of comparison.

Public opinion must also be studied. It would be useful to document how many women would prefer to give birth in a hospital setting or an alternative setting, and how many have a preference for a particular caregiver or combination of caregivers (obstetricians, midwives, general practitioners). It is clear that many midwives believe that a majority of expectant women would prefer the services of a midwife to other caregivers, provided that midwifery was legally recognized and offered by qualified midwives. A community midwife lamented this gap between existing clienteles and what could be achieved if midwifery were established in British Columbia: "There is such a small percentage of women with access to midwifery care. If midwifery was legalized and midwives were in the mainstream, 80 per cent of the population would use midwives. I think that consumer support is the only way." Survey research would be useful in generating measures of public opinion (see Greater Vancouver Regional District 1993). These surveys could be supplemented by in-depth interviews about particular preferences and the logic underlying respondents' opinions. There is a need to explore earlier suggestions of substantial challenges to physicians' authority in certain areas of health care.

A number of reports have favoured the legal recognition of midwifery practice and the provision of a variety of settings for practice. The Quebec Social Affairs and Family Council, an advisory body, recently recommended that pilot projects be undertaken in a variety of settings (Pelletier 1988, 43). Not surprisingly, efforts to reintroduce midwifery in Quebec generated considerable and sometimes outspoken dissent on the part of medical association representatives.

BIRTHING CENTRES AND WOMEN'S CLINICS

The introduction of alternative birth centres (ABCs) as a compromise between domiciliary birth settings and obstetrical wards is one example of innovation that rests, in part, on consumer demand. This apparently neat equation of birth innovations and public demand does not take into account the historical rivalry between various professional and non-professional associations (Freidson 1972; Mitford 1992). It also must address evidence that ABCs do not in fact significantly alter the incidence of obstetrical interventions.

DeVries contends that the apparent freedom accorded parturient women in ABCs is used to consolidate the power of the birth centre staff. Notwithstanding the homelike decor and nods toward unmedicated births, where possible, ABCs are characterized by unjustifiably high rates of invasive treatment, including analgesia, anaesthesia, episiotomy, and forceps delivery (DeVries 1980). DeVries (1984, 98) cites one study that documented a transfer rate of 46 per cent of patients from an alternative birth centre to a conventional labour and delivery suite. A documentary on home birth in the United States indicated that between 20 and 50 per cent of women entering an ABC will be transferred to operating rooms for a forceps delivery, caesarean section, electronic fetal monitoring, and so forth (CBS News 1982). Establishing birthing rooms in hospitals is another method of adapting settings to consumer demand. One difficulty that has been remarked on, however, is that in some hospitals the birthing rooms account for only a small proportion – in some cases as low as 3 per cent – of all births in hospital (Anonymous 1984, 14).

Some observers disagree that ABCs are in the best interest of pregnant women and infants. The growth of birth centres is tied to the professional interest of nurse-midwives, long subordinated to doctors' control through denial of hospital privileges and inadequate back-up services. Thus, hospital settings and birth centres pose disadvantages to pregnant women, although evidence on this point is not well substantiated and is at times contradictory. Rothman (1983) acknowledges that women giving birth in ABCs tend to be satisfied with their experience, and she appears to have a blind spot with respect to the limitations of home birth arrangements. There is evidence favourable to alternative birth centres. The transfer rate in a maternity centre in New York City is approximately 15 per cent, and most of the transfers are not for emergencies but rather for failure to progress in labour (ABC 1986). It has also been suggested that ABCs are less expensive to consumers and the state, and promote the safety of infants and mothers (Lubic 1983). Indeed, Lubic (1992) strongly endorses the work of family-oriented birth centres.

Another point of concern arises from the failure to establish out-of-hospital birthing centres. The recent denial of government funding to a Toronto-based group was ostensibly based on the lack of physician support for such a centre. An earlier proposal to develop an out-of-hospital clinic in Vancouver was not accepted by a federal funding agency. It was suggested that the lack of support for the clinic among physicians was a factor in rejecting the proposal. The resistance to such centres thus involves a measure of self-interest among more established institutional staff and professsions (Lubic 1983). It is important that ABCs be assessed in terms of who decides how birth is to be managed – the protocols for care, access of various caregivers, and expectant mothers' choices. DeVries's reservations – and he is not alone – provide a useful caution against innovations that are seemingly progressive but in fact reconsolidate professional power.

WOMEN'S CLINICS

A related initiative involves the use of women's clinics, which would provide a variety of health services for women, including maternity care. Currently, there is an attempt to develop such a clinic in Vancouver. Other models exist in the British National Health Service. In such clinics women are seen as "well" and not automatically as "sick." However, these clinics do not offer maternity services (Gardner 1981). These initiatives can be linked with the notions that women are to be cared for by women, and that available technology and knowledge can be applied in a setting conducive to the collective interests of women clients and practitioners. Services concerning obstetrics and gynecology would not be fragmented, and resources could be centralized. The women's clinic appears to be a reshaping of the former "community of women."

CONCLUSION

The initiatives of nurse-midwives and community midwives are far from a passing fashion, and should be taken seriously as instances of resistance and innovation in the interests of women and, more generally, of parents and health-care practitioners. In contrast to the stereotype of midwives as irresponsible and hazardous, and to the uncritical celebration of community midwifery as a service to women, this study underlines the differences between community midwives in various aspects of their work. Some are more willing than others to transfer women from home to hospital, to maintain thorough charts and other documentation, and to balance safe standards of practice against clients' wishes. Midwifery practice thus appears as a complex undertaking that has a collective base but is also rooted in some degree of idiosyncracy and disagreement over practices and the implications of legalizing and formalizing those practices.

A second contribution by midwives is their abiding interest in ensuring maternal and infant safety. My study and other studies of autonomous midwives provide some evidence in support of the safety of domiciliary midwifery and out-of-hospital settings, such as ABCs. These results are linked with a number of published articles and monographs from Holland, the United States, France, and England that report favourable birth outcomes in certain out-of-hospital settings.

On the basis of research reports published outside of Canada, and in the light of nurse-midwifery initiatives such as the Low-Risk Clinic and the Midwives' Project established at the Grace Hospital in Vancouver, it is argued that nurse-midwives have provided high-quality care in hospital settings. Moreover, some believe that midwives can preserve their philosophy of compassionate and skilled care within hospital settings (Brennan and Heilman 1977).

Historical and crosscultural sources have been set in the context of gender-related struggles over childbirth as a woman's process, a community event, and a profession. It is suggested that contemporary community midwives have attempted to rekindle an ancient tradition of women caring for women and to resist modern attempts to "commodify" childbirth in the general interests of men. The control of childbirth and of human reproduction generally can be seen as a symbolic expression of male dominance in childbirth and in medical research and practice. It is suggested that these struggles are not simply about "men versus women," however. Some men have been active in supporting more autonomous midwifery practice and its legalization, and women practitioners have been of service to women giving birth. The crux of the midwifery debate is therefore not reducible to gender, just as it is not reducible to class relations or to biology.

The research also raises serious questions about who sets the agenda for women's reproductive choices. This issue carries tremendous significance for women's rights in law, and has been addressed by several feminist writers concerned about the control of reproduction (Oakley 1980; O'Brien 1981; Stanworth 1987). The nature of state mediation is central to an understanding of the midwifery debate in Canada and in other countries. The replacement of community control over childbirth was made possible only through substantial powers of sanction and subsidization through the state. The tangible effects of facilitating hospital construction and medical and nursing education, and of applying criminal and quasi-criminal prosecution to rival health practitioners, served to consolidate medical dominance in health services. An important qualification to this instrumentalist approach is that clients also have powers to complain about unsatisfactory practices to medical and nursing colleges. Clients may also initiate civil actions alleging malpractice against physicians or nurses, and lobby state officials for improved health services. Furthermore, criminal actions against community midwives have not been used routinely, nor are they always successful. Like chiropractors (Mills and Larsen 1981, 237; Eni 1991), community midwives have increased in number and gained in official recognition despite the resistance of the medical profession.

Theories of the state have been critically assessed with respect to lobbying by community midwives and nurse-midwives. The structuralist perspective is useful in appreciating the relative autonomy of the state and the efforts of state agents to consolidate professional power and to "commodify" social relations in the interests of capital. The limits of the structuralist approach become apparent in the cultural pressures to resist statism and to preserve folk customs and civil liberties.

The status of modern midwifery in the Canadian provinces discussed herein becomes understandable in terms of the historical development of midwifery, from folk customs to professional practice, and in terms of the movement of the state as a mediator of long-standing conflicts between midwives, other practitioners, supply companies, and consumers. There is an enduring quality to midwifery practice, yet it becomes evident that the state has acted to constrain midwifery initiatives even as it helps to establish them. Again, this reflects the contradictory pressures on the state from outside and inside in formulating health-care policy.

The strong conflict between medical practitioners and midwives has its roots in the economic status secured by physicians. And it is clear that physicians are unlikely to endorse the introduction of other practitioners unless there is some material advantage to the profession – for example, if midwives are a source of referrals to physicians, or if the management of uncomplicated deliveries is not financially attractive to physicians.

The economic dimension in health care requires an appreciation of methods by which competitors can be constrained or eliminated when they attempt to provide health services: "Of course professional regulation can be used punitively by a dominant group of providers to discipline or suppress potential competitors. A policy of encouraging competitive forms of delivery which pose a real threat to 'mainstream' care markets must therefore include some monitoring and control of the professional self-regulatory process" (Evans 1984, 345).

The sphere of law is pertinent to this conflict. Community midwives practising in violation of the Medical Practitioners Act (in British Columbia) have been greatly constrained in establishing institutional supports for their work, most notably an out-of-hospital clinic or midwifery centre. While there have been only a few prosecutions of community midwives under the statute, and then only after an infant death following an attempted home delivery, more subtle constraints on autonomous midwifery practice are operating. These constraints have not been diminished greatly through the modern midwifery movement in Canada, despite the tension between the civil liberties of individuals versus the prohibitory powers of the state over human conduct. The restricted use of law reflects, among other things, the general safety of infants and mothers in the great majority of home births documented here and in jurisdictions other than Canada. It also may reflect the custom of women assisting women in childbirth. Sumner (1960) contended that folkways were powerful norms that influenced the nature of social life, and the nature of legal regulation of social life.

As has been suggested earlier, the collision of these perspectives has not produced a very robust defence of midwifery in Canada. The state has reacted by proceeding cautiously to favour midwifery (usually under the direction and supervison of medical or nursing personnel), or by not establishing midwifery services except in remote areas. It appears that a blend of structural constraints and human agency is evident in the limited restructuring of maternity services provided by midwives. This represents not an isolated instance of restricted social change, but rather the continuing role of the state in rationalizing social conflicts. That role involves the sub-sidization of orthodox health services and supplies and, occasionally, the deployment of criminal law personnel to repress practices that are seen as dangerous.

It is suggested that the Canadian state is not simply an instrument of a particular class or dominant grouping, nor is its health policy clearly tied to a specific economic base. A structuralist approach seems most appropriate in order to understand continuing patterns of occupational stratification (by gender and class), but this is a modified structuralism that must account for the role of human agency. Lobbying by nurse-midwives and nurses' associations, con-sumer demand, and the individual efforts of various officials have encouraged a growing recognition of midwifery services by the state and are therefore integral to the midwifery debate.

Understanding midwifery requires an appreciation of the forces that oppose its implementation as a self-governing profession in Canada. Despite some differences of opinion in the more established professions of medicine and nursing, there has generally been little encouragement of midwifery by national or provincial medical or nursing associations. Those associations that have expressed support for midwifery have almost invariably expressed caveats about home birth and other facets of what is seen by Canadian midwives as independent practice. Opposition can take many forms: the very negative pronouncements against midwives in Quebec (Bantey 1989; Dunn 1993) and Alberta (including an explicit ban on physicians' assisting midwives in home births in Alberta), or the seemingly more reasoned arguments that midwifery can be readily absorbed into nursing practice. Materially, the economic power of these professions seems to be threatened by the recognition of another health specialty in the area of obstetrics.

The discourse about midwifery is in large part mired in discussions of whether midwifery is really necessary, and if so, how it ought to be implemented. As noted above, midwives are being asked to take a considerable portion of water with their wine. The discourse nevertheless rests on a number of fundamental contradictions: first, how women can be denied options for birth when women are the carriers and deliverers of children; second, questions surrounding unfair restraint on freedom of choice in a democratic society; and, third, continuing concerns over the lack of intimacy and undue interference in childbirth on the part of many established professions and institutions. Difficulties women experience in arranging for VBAC deliveries are one example of limited options in birth; so also is the current statistic that 22 per cent of women currently giving birth in British Columbia are delivered by caesarean section.

The discourse against midwifery, once hegemonic in Canada, is challenged at every step on principle, and usually with supportive data on hand. This challenge to opponents of midwifery is rendered more acute by Canada's anomalous failure to legally recognize midwifery, a string of official recommendations to legalize midwives, and the example of a minority of provinces that have begun to establish midwifery as a distinct profession. The legacy of the community midwives, of the Grace Hospital Low-Risk and Midwifery programs in the 1980s and 1990s, and of Inuit midwives working with other practitioners in Povungnituk (Arctic Quebec) lend further weight to the viability of midwifery. The argument for midwifery is not set against the appropriate use of technology in obstetrics, but against an overshadowing of midwifery skills – and, not least of all, women's abilities to give birth – by an ideology of "machine-minding." Ironically, as medical and social science knowledge increase in the sphere of reproduction, there is a considerable body of literature that draws our attention to the limits of routine monitoring of birth, and many conventions surrounding birth as a medical event.

It may be anticipated that state initiatives will involve a gradual expansion of the qualified midwife's role and the legalization of midwifery as an occupation separate from medicine. This expansion of the midwife's role may stem from a number of pressures. These include the international and provincial lobbying for reinstatement of the midwife, research that supports the safety of qualified midwifery attendance (in hospital, clinic, and domiciliary practice), and the state's need to rationalize and legitimate health-care policies for consumers. It may be that the provincial governments in Canada will differ in the pace and scope of legalization. This may reflect differences in political lobbying, consumer preferences, and the sensitivity of the government of the day to women's issues. The historical specificity of the state – whether local, provincial, or national – remains an important dimension in the evolution of midwifery practice and its future development. The historical development and extension of state powers in Canada has hindered the growth of autonomous midwifery practice. State control in the sphere of birthing cannot be separated from cultural stereotypes of birth as dangerous (and therefore in need of professional management), and the long-standing fear of women's self-determination as individuals and as a community. In this sense, contemporary midwives are struggling against a state structure and a cultural heritage that are intolerant of such concerted efforts to wrest control from the medical and nursing professions. Midwives are also struggling with the tangible discretionary powers of ministry officials, which may be applied to scrutinize midwifery practice and only reluctantly to promote its development other than through the hierarchy of medicine, or the ranking of professional over layperson (see Neilans 1992).

There are variations and contradictions in provincial policies, in the decisions of judicial and quasi-judicial bodies, in midwifery practice, and in public support, to name only a few. These variations undermine a monolithic portrait of the total domination of women's choices. Thus, contradiction and paradox are evident in the current structure of maternity and infant care in Canada. In the historical treatment of midwives and the near-elimination of the autonomous community midwife in Canada, powerful structural forces restrict women's self-determination, even when such self-determination and community support can be shown to be advantageous for women and their children. It is clear that the "ancient office" of the midwife is not well served by repressive legal enactments and policies. Under such conditions midwifery may endure, but it will not flourish. The struggle to broaden the range of choice for expectant mothers, and to reconstitute our modern communities along more intimate lines, remains at the heart of activism on behalf of midwives and their clients.

Glossary

The following terms are commonly used in maternity and infant care. More comprehensive glossaries are available in a variety of books including Margaret Jensen, Ralph Benson, and Irene Bobak, *Maternity Care: The Nurse and the Family* (St. Louis: Mosby, 1979), and Roger Tonkin, *Child Health Profile: Birth Events and Infant Outcomes* (Vancouver: Hemlock Printers).

abortion   A spontaneous abortion is the expulsion of a non-viable fetus that occurs naturally. A therapeutic abortion is an intentional termination of a pregnancy under medical care.

afterbirth   The placenta and fetal membranes expelled after delivery of the child.

amniocentesis   A procedure used to assess fetal health and functioning whereby a needle is inserted through the woman's abdominal and uterine walls to obtain amniotic fluid.

analgesic   Any drug or agent that relieves pain.

Apgar score   A scale of measurement, developed by Dr. Beverly Apgar, by which a newborn's heart rate, respiration, muscle tone, reflex irritability, and skin colour are assessed. Assessments are conventionally made 1 minute, 5 minutes, and 10 (or 15) minutes after birth.

breech presentation   Buttocks and/or feet of the child are closest to the cervical opening, and are born first. Breech birth occurs in approximately 3 per cent of all deliveries. A complete breech occurs when buttocks, legs, and feet are presented simultaneously. A footling breech involves presentation of one or both feet. A frank breech involves the presentation of the buttocks, with hips flexed so that the baby's thighs are pressed against its stomach.

caesarean section   A surgical incision of the abdominal wall and uterus for delivery of the infant.

episiotomy   Surgical enlargement of the perineal area to facilitate delivery and avoid perineal lacerations.

intrapartum   During birth.

infant mortality rate   The number of deaths of infants under one year of age, excluding stillbirths, per one thousand live births.

lithotomy position   Delivery position in which the woman lies on her back with her knees flexed and her abducted thighs drawn toward her chest.

meconium aspiration syndrome   With fetal hypoxia (insufficient availability of oxygen to meet the infant's metabolic needs), the anal sphincter relaxes and meconium is released. Reflex grasping movements may draw meconium into the amniotic fluid and into the infant's bronchial tree, obstructing air flow after birth.

multigravida   A woman who has been pregnant two or more times.

multipara   A woman who has carried two or more pregnancies to viability, whether or not they ended in live births or stillbirths.

neonatal mortality rate   The number of neonatal deaths during the first twenty-eight days after delivery, excluding stillbirths, per one thousand live births.

perinatal mortality rate   The number of deaths of fetuses 20 or more weeks' gestation, plus the number of deaths of infants under seven days of age, per one thousand total births, expressed per one thousand live births.

perineum   The area between the anus and the external genitalia.

placenta previa   Abnormal implantation of the placenta in the lower uterine segment, resulting in the placenta's covering all or part of the cervical os (opening).

post-neonatal period   The period of infancy between 28 days and 365 days.

premature   Born after a gestation period of less than thirty-seven weeks.

prenatal period   The period of pregnancy between conception and the onset of labor.

primigravida   A woman who is pregnant for the first time.

primipara   A woman who has carried one pregnancy to viability, whether or not the child is born alive or stillborn.

quasi-criminal offence   An offence that is not a crime or misdemeanour, but that is in the nature of a crime, to which a penalty or forfeiture is attached.

retained placenta   That part of the placenta that is retained in the uterus after delivery.

Schultze   (Also known as "Schultze's mechanism.") Delivery of the placenta with the fetal surfaces (shiny in appearance) presenting. Also termed "shiny Schultze."

stillbirth rate   The number of fetal deaths based on weight (five hundred grams or more), or on gestation (usually twenty to twenty-eight weeks).

term   The time at which a pregnancy of normal length terminates (between thirty-seven and forty-two weeks).

Table of Cases

Bibliography

ABC News. 1986. Mary Rossi, speaking on *Nightline*, October.

Alternative Birth Crisis Coalition. 1984. "News Analysis – Canada: Midwives on Trial." *ABCC News* 111:3–4.

Anderson, Cheryl. 1986. "Midwifery and the Family Physician." *Canadian Family Physician* 32:11–15.

Andrews, Margaret. 1978–9. "Medical Attendance in Vancouver, 1886–1920." *B.C. Studies* 40:32–56.

Anisef, P., and P. Basson. 1979. "Institutionalization of a Profession: Comparison of British and American Midwifery." *Sociology of Work and Occupations* 6:353–72.

Annas, George. 1977. "Legal Aspects of Homebirths and other Childbirth Alternatives." In *Safe Alternatives in Childbirth*, edited by D. Stewart and L. Stewart. Marble Hill, Mo.: National Association of Parents and Professionals for Alternatives in Childbirth (NAPSAC).

– 1978. "Homebirth: Autonomy vs. Safety." *The Hastings Center Report*, 8:19–20.

Anonymous. 1981. "Grace Hospital, Doctor Faulted in Baby's Birth." *Vancouver Sun*, 7 April.

– 1984. "Nurse says Hospital Avoids Night Births." *Globe and Mail*.

– 1986. "International News." *Midwifery* 2:53.

– 1986a. "Midwife Crossroads." *Vancouver Sun*, 11 October.

– 1987. "Health Views." *Today's Health* (March) 62–3.

Archer, John, and Barbara Lloyd. 1985. *Gender*. Harmondsworth: Penguin.

Arms, Suzanne. 1977. *Immaculate Deception*. New York: Bantam Books.

Armstrong, Penny, and Sheryl Feldman. 1986. *A Midwife's Story*. Toronto: Fitzhenry and Whiteside.

Arney, William Ray. 1982. *Power and the Profession of Obstetrics*. Chicago: University of Chicago Press.

Asher, Arney. 1981. "Health Care in Israel: Political and Administrative Aspects." *International Political Science Review* 2:43–6.

Ashley, Jo Ann. 1980. "Power in Structured Misogyny: Implications for the Politics of Care." *Annals of Nursing Science* 2:3–22.

Askew, I., M. Carballo, S. Ritkin, and D. Saunders. 1989. *Policy Aspects of Community Participation in Maternal and Child Health and Family Planning Programmes*. Geneva: World Health Organization and United Nations Population Fund.

Association of Radical Midwives. 1986. *The Vision: Proposals for the Future of the Maternity Services*. Ormskirk: Association of Radical Midwives.

Babbie, Earl. 1979. *The Practice of Social Research*, 2d ed. Belmont: Wadsworth.

Backhouse, Constance. 1991. *Petticoats and Prejudice: Women and Law in Nineteenth-Century Canada*. Toronto: The Osgoode Society.

Badinter, Elisabeth. 1981. *The Myth of Motherhood: An Historical View of the Maternal Instinct*. London: Souvenir Press.

Bagnell, Kenneth. 1980. *The Little Immigrants: The Orphans Who Came to Canada*. Toronto: Macmillan.

Baker, Maureen. 1990. *Midwifery: A New Status*. Background paper for the Library of Parliament (BP-217E). Ottawa: Ministry of Supply and Services.

Balbus, Isaac D. 1978. "Commodity Form and Legal Form: An Essay on the 'Relative Autonomy' of the Law." In *The Sociology of Law: A Conflict Perspective*, edited by C. Reasons and R. Rich. Toronto: Butterworths.

Banks, Shelley. 1986. "Witness Backs Home Births." *Vancouver Sun*, 26 June.

Bantey, Ed. 1989. "Quebec Doctors Will Have to Deal with Midwife Issue." *The Gazette*, 16 April.

Barrington, Eleanor. 1985. *Midwifery Is Catching*. Toronto: NC Press.

Bastian, H. and P. Lancaster. 1990. *Home Births in Australia 1985–87*. Sydney: National Perinatal Statistics Unit.

Baum, Gregory. 1990. "The Postmodern Age." *Canadian Forum* (May) 5–7.

Begum, Ara, Iqbal Kabir, and Yasin Mollah. 1990. "The Impact of Training Traditional Birth Attendants in Improving MCH [Maternal and Child Health] Care in Rural Bangladesh." *Asia-Pacific Journal of Public Health* 4(2–3): 142–4.

Beirne, Piers, and Robert Sharlet, eds. 1980. *Paskukanis: Selected Writings on Marxism and Law*. London: Academic Press.

Beischer, Norman, and Eric Mackay. 1986. *Obstetrics and the Newborn: An Illustrated Textbook*, 2d ed. Sydney: W.B. Saunders.

Benedek, Thomas. 1977. "The Changing Relationship between Midwives and Physicians during the Renaissance." *Bulletin of the History of Medicine* 51:550–64.

Benoit, Cecilia. 1983. "Midwives and Healers: The Newfoundland Experience." *Healthsharing* (Winter) 22–6.

– 1988. "Traditional Midwifery Practice: The Limits of Occupational Autonomy." *Canadian Review of Sociology and Anthropology* 26:633–49.

– 1991. *Midwives in Passage: The Modernisation of Maternity Care*. St. John's: Institute of Social and Economic Research.

Ben-Yehuda, N. 1980. "The European Witch-Craze of the 14th to 17th Centuries: A Sociologist's Perspective." *American Journal of Sociology* 86:1–31.

Berton, Pierre. 1977. *The Dionne Years: A Thirties Melodrama*. Toronto: McClelland and Stewart.

Besharaw, A. 1985. "Jury Recommends Legalization, Recognition of Midwifery in Ontario." *Canadian Nurse* (September) 11.

Bhatia, S. 1981. "Traditional Childbirth Practices: Implications for a Rural MCH Program." *Studies in Family Planning* 12:66–74.

Biernacki, P., and D. Waldorf. 1981. "Snowball Sampling: Problems and Techniques of Chain Referral Sampling." *Sociological Methods and Research* 10:141–63.

Biggar, J. 1972. "When Midwives Were Witches ... White Ones of Course: A Look at Maternity Care in the Middle Ages." *Nursing Mirror and Midwives' Journal* 134:37–9.

Biggs, Lesley. 1983. "The Case of the Missing Midwives: A History of Midwifery in Ontario from 1795–1900." *Ontario History* 75:21–35.

– 1988. "The Profession of Chiropractic in Canada: Its Current Struggles and Future Prospects." In *Sociology of Health Care in Canada*, edited by B.S. Bolaria and H. Dickenson. Toronto: Harcourt Brace Jovanovich.

Bittman, S., and S. Rosenberg Zalk. 1978. *Expectant Fathers*. New York: Hawthorn.

Bohme, Gernot. 1984. "Midwifery as Science: An Essay on the Relation between Scientific and Everyday Knowledge." In *Society and Knowledge: Contemporary Perspectives in the Sociology of Knowledge*, edited by N. Stehr and V. Meja. New Brunswick, N.J.: Transaction Books.

Bolaria, B. Singh, and Peter Li, eds. 1988. *Racial Oppression in Canada*. Toronto: Garamond.

Bosk, C. 1979. *Forgive and Remember: Managing Medical Failure*. Chicago: University of Chicago Press.

Boston Women's Health Collective. 1992. *The New Our Bodies, Ourselves*. New York: Simon and Schuster.

Bourque, P. 1980. "Proof of the Cause of Death in a Prosecution for Criminal Negligence Causing Death." *Criminal Law Quarterly* 22:334–43.

Brack, Datha. 1976. "Displaced: The Midwife by the Male Physician." *Women and Health* 1:18–24.

Bradley, C.F., S.E. Ross, A.C. Rutter, J.M. Warnyca, and J.M. Cockling. 1978. *Perinatal Health for the City*. Vancouver: Vancouver Perinatal Health Project.

Bradley-Low, A. 1984. "Observations on Midwifery and Maternity Care in Japan." *Issue* 5:13–14.

Brendsel, C., G. Peterson, and L. Mehl. 1979. "Episiotomy: Facts, Fictions, Figures, and Alternatives." In *Compulsory Hospitalization or Freedom of Choice in Childbirth*, vol. 1, edited by D. Stewart and L. Stewart. Marble Hill, Mo.: NAPSAC.

Brennan, Barbara, and Joan Heilman. 1977. *The Complete Book of Midwifery*. New York: E.P. Dutton.

British Columbia. 1992. *Selected Vital Statistics and Health Status Indicators: 120th Annual Report 1991*. Victoria: Division of Vital Statistics.

Brockman, Joan. 1992. "'Resistance by the Club' to the Feminization of the Legal Profession." *Canadian Journal of Law and Society* 7:47–86.

Brook, P. 1980. "Midwives and Medicine." *The Magazine* (May) 18:6–8.

Brooks, C. 1980. "Social, Economic, and Biologic Correlates of Infant Mortality in City Neighbourhoods." *Journal of Health and Social Behavior* 21:2–11.

Brooks, Tonya, and Linda Bennett. 1976. *Giving Birth at Home*. Curritos, Calif.: Association for Childbirth at Home International.

Buckley, Suzann. 1979. "Ladies or Midwives? Efforts to Reduce Infant and Maternal Mortality." In *A Not Unreasonable Claim: Women and Reform in Canada, 1880s–1920s*, edited by L. Kealey. Toronto: The Women's Press.

Burke, Peter. 1981. "People's History or Total History." In *People's History and Socialist Theory*, edited by R. Samuel. London: Routledge and Kegan Paul.

Burnett III, C., et al. 1980. "Home Delivery and Neonatal Mortality in North Carolina." *Journal of the American Medical Association* 244:2741–5.

Burris, H.L. 1967 *Medical Saga: The Burris Clinic and Early Pioneers*. Kamloops: Mitchell Press.

Burtch, Brian. 1987. "Community Midwives and State Measures: The New Midwifery in Canada." *Contemporary Crises* 10:131–49.

– 1987a. "Midwifery Practice and State Regulation: A Sociological Approach." PH.D. thesis, University of British Columbia.

– 1988. "Midwives and the State: The New Midwifery in Canada." In *Gender and Society: Creating a Canadian Women's Sociology*, edited by A. McLaren. Toronto: Copp Clark Pitman.

– 1988a. "Promoting Midwifery, Prosecuting Midwives: The State and the Midwifery Movement in Canada." In *Sociology of Health Care in Canada*, edited by B.S. Bolaria and H. Dickenson. Toronto: Harcourt Brace Jovanovich.

– 1992. *The Sociology of Law: Critical Approaches to Social Control*. Toronto: HBJ Holt Canada.

Burtch, Brian, A. Wachtel, and C. Pitcher-LaPrairie. 1985. "Marriage Preparation, Separation, Conciliation and Divorce: Findings from the Images of Law Study." *Canadian Journal of Family Law* 4:369–84.

Buss, F. 1980. *La Partera: Story of a Midwife*. Ann Arbor: University of Michigan Press.

Butani, P., and E. Hadnett. 1980. "Mothers' Perceptions of Their Labor Experiences." *Maternal and Child Nursing Journal* 9:73–82.

Butter, Irene, and Bonnie Kay. 1988. "State Laws and the Practice of Lay Midwifery." *American Journal of Public Health* 78:1161–9.

Cameron, Anne. 1982. *The Journey*. New York: Avon.

Cameron, J., E. Chase, and S. O'Neal. 1979. "Home Birth in Salt Lake County, Utah." *American Journal of Public Health* 69:716–17.

Campbell, R., and A. Macfarlane. 1987. *Where to Be Born? The Debate and the Evidence*. Oxford: National Perinatal Epidemiology Unit.

Campbell, Rona. 1992. "Review of Marjorie Tew, *Safer Childbirth*." MIDIRS *Midwifery Digest* 2:364.

Campbell, Marie. 1946. *Folks Do Get Born*. New York: Rinehart and Co.

Campbell, S. 1982. "Midwives United: The Midwives Alliance of North America." *Mothering* 24:75–6.

Canadian Broadcasting Corporation. 1981. David Cayley, "Midwifery in Canada: Part IV." *Morningside*.

Canadian Confederation of Midwives. 1992. *Annual Report*. Toronto: Canadian Confederation of Midwives.

Canadian Press. 1976. "Parents Must Decide on Home Childbirth." *The Province*, 26 August.

– 1987. "Birthing Care Gets a 'Satisfactory' Rating." *Vancouver Sun*, 3 April.

Caputo, T., M. Kennedy, C. Reasons, and A. Brannigan, eds. 1989. *Law and Society: A Critical Perspective*. Toronto: Harcourt Brace Jovanovich.

Cartwright, A. 1979. *The Dignity of Labour? A Study of Childbearing and Induction*. London: Tavistock.

Carty, E., S. Effer, D. Farquharson, J. King, A. Rice, D. Tier, L. Wetherston, and B. Wittmann. 1984. *The Low-Risk Clinic: Family Care Based on the Midwifery Model, 1981–1984*. Vancouver: Shaughnessy Hospital Education Services and School of Nursing, University of British Columbia.

Carver, C. 1981. "The Deliverers: A Woman Doctor's Reflections on Medical Socialization." In *Childbirth: Alternatives to Medical Control*, edited by S. Romalis. Austin: University of Texas Press.

Cave, C. 1978. "Social Characteristics of Natural Childbirth Users and Non-Users." *American Journal of Public Health* 68:898–900.

Chambliss, W. 1986. "On Lawmaking." In *The Social Basis of Law*, edited by S. Brickey and E. Comack. Toronto: Garamond.

Chen, P.C.Y. 1977. "Incorporating the Traditional Birth Attendant into the Health Team." *Tropical and Geographic Medicine* 29:192–6.

– 1978. "Reasons Underlying the Maternal Choice of Midwives in Rural Malaysia." *Medical Journal of Malaysia* 32:200–5.

Chodorow, Nancy. 1971. "Being and Doing: A Cross-Cultural Examination of the Socialization of Males and Females." In *Women in Sexist Society:*

Studies in Power and Powerlessness, edited by Vivian Gornick and Barbara Goran. New York: Mentor.

Christie, Nils. 1978. "Conflicts as Property." In *The Sociology of Law*, edited by C. Reasons and R. Rich. Toronto: Butterworths.

Cobb, Ann Kuckelman. 1981. "Incorporation and Change: The Case of the Midwife in the United States." *Medical Anthropology* 5:73–88.

Coburn, David. 1980. "Patients' Rights: A New Deal in Health Care." *Canadian Forum* (May) 14–18.

Coburn, David, George Torrance, and Joseph Kaufert. 1983. "Medical Dominance in Canada in Historical Perspective: The Rise and Fall of Medicine?" *International Journal of Health Services* 13:407–32.

Coburn, Judi. 1974. "'I See and Am Silent': A Short History of Nursing in Ontario." In *Women at Work: Ontario, 1850–1930*, edited by Janice Acton, Penny Goldsmith, and Bonnie Shepard. Toronto: Canadian Women's Educational Press.

Cohen, Nancy. 1991. *Open Season: A Survival Guide for Natural Childbirth and Vaginal Birth After Caesarean Section in the 90s*. New York: Bergin and Garvey.

Cohen, Nancy, and Lois J. Estner. 1983. *Silent Knife: Caesarean Prevention and Vaginal Birth after Caesarean (VBAC)*. South Hadley: Bergin and Garvey Publishers.

Cohen, Stanley. 1985. *Visions of Social Control*. London: Polity Press.

Colette. 1979. "The Patriarch." In *The Rainy Moon and Other Stories*, translated by Antonia White. Harmondsworth: Penguin.

College of Nurses of Ontario. 1983. "Guidelines for Registered Nurses Providing Care to Individuals and Families Seeking Alternatives to Childbirth in a Hospital Setting." Toronto: College of Nurses of Ontario (typescript).

CBS News. 1982. "Home Births." *60 Minutes*, 21 March.

CBS Reports. 1981. "Nurse ... Where Are You?" 28 May.

Conklin, Nancy Faires, Brenda McCallum, and Marcia Wade. 1983. *The Culture of Southern Black Women: Approaches and Materials*. University of Alabama: Archive of American Minority Cultures and Women's Studies Program.

Connell, D.J.R. 1980. "Obstetric Anesthetist's Views Should Be Heard." *Vancouver Sun*, 27 August.

Converse, Thomas A., Richard S. Buker and Richard V. Lee. 1973. "Hutterite Midwifery." *American Journal of Obstetrics and Gynecology* 116:719–25.

Cook, Ramsay, and Wendy Mitchinson, eds. 1976. *The Proper Sphere: Women's Place in Canadian Society*. Toronto: Oxford University Press.

Cooke, Dave. 1984. "Government Should Recognize Midwifery." *NDP News* (4 December) 30.

Corea, Gene. 1985. *The Mother Machine: Reproductive Technologies from Artificial Insemination to Artificial Wombs*. New York: Harper and Row.

Cosbie, W.G. 1969. *The History of the Society of Obstetricians and Gynaecologists of Canada*. N.p., n.p.

Cosminsky, Sheila. 1976. "Cross-Cultural Perspectives on Midwifery." In *Medical Anthropology: Proceedings of the Ninth International Congress of Anthropological and Ethnological Sciences Held in Chicago, 1973*, edited by Francis Grollig and Harold Haley. Paris and the Hague: Mouton.

– 1977. "Childbirth and Midwifery on a Guatemalan Finca." *Medical Anthropology* 3:69–104.

Cotterrell, Roger. 1984. *The Sociology of Law: An Introduction*. Toronto: Butterworths.

Coughlin, Richard J. 1965. "Pregnancy and Birth in Vietnam." In *Southeast Asia Birth Customs: Three Studies in Human Reproduction*, edited by D. Hart et al. New Haven: Human Relations Area Files Press.

Cox, Sue. 1991. "Dissenting Voices: New Reproductive Technology and Feminist Analyses." MA thesis, Simon Fraser University.

Crawford, Robert. 1980. "Healthism and the Medicalization of Everyday Life." *International Journal of Health Services* 10:365–88.

Creese, Gillian, and Veronica Strong-Boag, eds. 1992. *British Columbia Reconsidered: Essays on Women*. Vancouver: Press Gang.

Cruz, V. da. 1969. *Balliere's Midwives' Dictionary*, 5th ed. London: Balliere Tindall and Cassell.

CSP Editors. 1982. "Birth Rights: Consumerism in Health Care." *Critical Social Policy* 2:62–5.

Cutshall, Pat. 1987. "Midwifery Revisited." *RNABC News* (July–August) 23.

Daly, Mary. 1978. *Gyn/Ecology: The Metaethics of Radical Feminism*. Boston: Beacon Press.

Damstra-Wijmenga, S.M. 1984. "Home Confinement: The Positive Results in Holland." *Journal of the Royal College of General Practitioners* 34:425–31.

Danzinger, Sandra. 1979. "Treatment of Women in Childbirth – Implications for Family Beginnings." *American Journal of Public Health* 69:895–902.

Davis, Elizabeth. 1981. *A Guide to Midwifery: Heart and Hands*. Santa Fe: John Muir Publications.

Davis-Floyd, R. 1990. "The Role of Obstetrical Rituals in the Resolution of Cultural Anomaly." *Social Science and Medicine* 31(2): 175–89.

Decker, Francis, Margaret Fougberg, and Mary Ronayne. 1978. *Pemberton: The History of a Settlement*, 2d ed. (rev.). Pemberton, B.C.: Pemberton Pioneer Women.

Devine, Cindy. 1981. "Childbirth Surrounded by Myths, Lack of Medical Information." *Network of Saskatchewan Women* 1:6–7.

Devitt, Neal. 1979. "Hospital Birth vs. Home Birth: The Scientific Facts, Past and Present." In *Compulsory Hospitalization or Freedom of Choice in*

Childbirth, vol. 2, edited by David Stewart and Lee Stewart. Marble Hill, Mo.: NAPSAC.

DeVries, Raymond. 1980. "The Alternative Birth Center: Option or Cooption?" *Women and Health* 5:47–60.

– 1984. "'Humanizing' Childbirth: The Discovery and Implementation of Bonding Theory." *International Journal of Health Services* 14:89–104.

– 1985. *Regulating Birth: Midwives, Medicine, and the Law*. Philadelphia: Temple University Press.

de Wolff, Alice. 1990. "Index on Canadian Women." *Canadian Forum* (December) 32.

Divorky, Diane. 1981. "Resistance: Midwives Moving into Physician Territory." *Sacramento Bee*, 29 April.

Dobbin, M. 1990. "Laying Waste to Saskatchewan Democracy." *Canadian Forum* (April) 8–13.

Dole, Gertrude. 1974. "The Marriages of Pacho: A Woman's Life among the Amahuaca." In *Many Sisters: Women in Cross-Cultural Perspective*, edited by C. Mattiasson. New York: The Free Press.

Donegan, Jane. 1978. *Women and Men Midwives*. Westport: Greenwood Press.

Donnison, Jean. 1977. *Midwives and Medical Men: A History of Interpersonal Rivalries and Women's Rights*. London: Heinemann.

– 1981. "The Development of the Occupation of Midwife: A Comparative View." In *Midwifery Is a Labour of Love*, Midwifery Task Force and British Columbia Association of Midwives. Vancouver: Maternal Health Society.

– 1988. *Midwives and Medical Men: A History of the Struggle for the Control of Childbirth* (rev. ed.). London: Historical Publications.

Donzelot, Jacques. 1979. *The Policing of Families*. New York: Pantheon.

Doyal, Lesley (with Imogen Pennel). 1981. *The Political Economy of Health*. Boston: South End Press.

Drachman, Virginia. 1979. "The Loomis Trial: Social Mores and Obstetrics in the Mid-Nineteenth Century." In *Health Care in America: Essays in Social History*, edited by S. Reverby and D. Rosner. Philadelphia: Temple University Press.

Dunn, Kate. 1993. "Legalize Midwifery Now, MD Urges Quebec: Practice Is Safe, so Pilot Projects Are Unnecessary: McGill Researcher." *The Gazette*, 5 March.

Eaton, Mary. 1990. "Lesbians and the Law." In *Lesbians in Canada*, edited by S. Stone. Toronto: Between the Lines.

Edge, Marc. 1986. "Midwives May Face Jail in Dec[ember]." *Vancouver Sun*, 10 October.

Edwards, Margot, and Mary Waldorf. 1984. *Reclaiming Birth: History and Heroines of American Childbirth Reform*. Trumansburg, N.Y.: The Crossing Press.

Ehrenreich, Barbara, and Deirdre English. 1973. *Witches, Midwives and Nurses.* Old Westbury, N.Y.: The Feminist Press.

Ehrenreich, Barbara, and John Ehrenreich. 1978. "Medicine and Social Control." In *The Cultural Crisis of Modern Medicine*, edited by J. Ehrenreich. New York: Monthly Review Press.

Eichler, Margrit, and Jeanne LaPointe. 1985. *On the Treatment of the Sexes in Research.* Ottawa: Social Sciences and Humanities Research Council of Canada.

Eickelman, Christine. 1984. *Women and Community in Oman.* New York: New York University Press.

Eisenstein, Zillah. 1981. *The Radical Future of Liberal Feminism.* New York: Longman.

Elliott, Jean, and Augie Fleras. 1992. *Unequal Relations: An Introduction to Race and Ethnic Dynamics in Canada.* Toronto: Prentice-Hall.

Eni, Godwin. 1991. "Chiropractic in British Columbia: Sociopolitical and Clinical Considerations for Strategic Planning." *Journal of Manipulative and Physiological Therapeutics* 14:29–37.

Enkin, Murray, Marc Keirse, and Iain Chalmers. 1989. *A Guide to Effective Care in Pregnancy and Childbirth.* Oxford: Oxford University Press.

Evans, Robert. 1984. *Strained Mercy: The Economics of Health Care in Canada.* Toronto: Butterworths.

Ewan, Stuart. 1972. "Charlie Manson and the Family: Authoritarianism and the Bourgeois Conception of 'Utopia': Some Thoughts on Charlie Manson and the Fantasy of the *Id.*" *Working Paper in Cultural Studies*, vol. 3. Birmingham: Centre for Contemporary Cultural Studies.

Epstein, Samuel. 1979. *The Politics of Cancer.* Garden City: Anchor Books.

Ericson, Richard, and Patricia Baranek. 1982. *The Ordering of Justice: A Study of Accused Persons as Dependants in the Criminal Process.* Toronto: University of Toronto Press.

Feyerabend, Paul. 1980. "Democracy, Elitism, and Scientific Method." *Inquiry* 23:3–18.

Field, Peggy Anne. 1991. "Midwifery in Canada." *Northwest Territories Registered Nurses Association Newsletter* (November) 4–6.

Fine, Bob. 1984. *Democracy and the Rule of Law: Liberal Ideals and Marxist Critiques.* London: Pluto Press.

Flint, Caroline. 1986. *Sensitive Midwifery.* London: Heinemann.

– 1986a. "Should Midwives Train as Florists?" *Nursing Times*, 12 February.

– 1991. "Continuity of Care Provided by a Team of Midwives – The Know Your Midwife Scheme." In *Midwives, Research and Childbirth*, vol. 2, edited by S. Robinson and A. Thomson. London: Chapman and Hall.

Forrest, Mary. 1978–79. "Natural Childbirth: Rights and Liabilities of the Parties." *Journal of Family Law* 17:309–32.

Foucault, Michel. 1973. *The Birth of the Clinic: An Archaeology of Medical Perception*. New York: Vintage.

– 1977. *Discipline and Punish: The Birth of the Prison*. New York: Vintage.

Francome, Colin. 1986. "The Fashion for Caesareans." *New Society*, 17 January.

Freemont Birth Collective. 1977. "Lay Midwifery – Still an 'Illegal' Profession." *Women and Health* 2:19–27.

Freidson, Eliot. 1970. *Profession of Medicine*. New York: Dodd, Mead.

– 1970a. *Professional Dominance: The Social Structure of Medical Care*. Chicago: Aldine.

– 1972. "The Organization of Medical Practice." In *Handbook of Medical Sociology*, edited by H. Freeman, S. Levine, and L. Reeder. Englewood Cliffs, N.J.: Prentice-Hall.

Friedenberg, Edgar. 1980. *Deference to Authority: The Case of Canada*. New York: Sharpe.

Frontier Nursing Service. 1975. *Medical Directives for the Use of the Nursing Staff of the Frontier Nursing Service Inc.*, 7th ed. (rev.). Wendover, Ky.: Frontier Nursing Service.

Fry, Hedy. 1987. "Home Birth: Safety Comes First." *The Province*, 22 November.

Fuentes, Annette, and Barbara Ehrenreich. 1991. *Women in the Global Factory*. Boston: South End Press.

Gahagan, Alvine Cyr. 1979. *Yes, Father: Pioneer Nursing in Alberta*. Manchester, N.H.: Hammer Publications.

Garcia, Jo, and Sally Garforth. 1991. "Midwifery Policies and Policy-Making." In *Midwives, Research and Childbirth*, vol. 3, edited by S. Robinson and A. Thomson. London: Chapman and Hall.

Gardner, Katy. 1981. "Well Woman Clinics: A Positive Approach to Women's Health." In *Women, Health and Reproduction*, edited by H. Roberts. London: Routledge and Kegan Paul.

Gaskin, Ina May. 1978. "Spiritual Midwifery on the Farm in Summertown, Tennessee." *Birth and the Family Journal* 5(2), 102–4.

– 1978a. *Spiritual Midwifery* (rev. ed.). Summertown, Tenn.: The Book Publishing Co.

– 1988. "Midwifery Re-Invented." In *The Midwife Challenge*, edited by S. Kitzinger, 42–60. London: Pandora.

Gaskin, Ina, and Stephen Gaskin. 1979. "Birth in a Community Where Home Is the Norm and Hospital the Exception." In *Compulsory Hospitalization or Freedom of Choice in Childbirth*, vol. 3, edited by D. Stewart and L. Stewart. Marble Hill, Mo.: NAPSAC.

Gay, Peter. 1970. *The Enlightenment: An Interpretation. Volume II: The Science of Freedom*. London: Weidenfeld and Nicholson.

Gelis, Jacques. 1991. *History of Childbirth: Fertility, Pregnancy and Birth in Early Modern Europe*, translated by Rosemary Morris. Boston: Northeastern University Press.

Ghosh-Ray, G.C., et al. 1980. "An Integrated Pain Relief Service for Labour: Co-operation between Obstetricians, Anesthetists, and Midwives." *Anaesthesia* 35:510–13.

Gibbon, Jan, and Mary Matthewson. 1947. *Three Centuries of Canadian Nursing*. Toronto: Macmillan.

Giddens, Anthony. 1982. *Profiles and Critiques in Social Theory*. Berkeley: University of California Press.

Ginzberg, Ruth. 1989. "Uncovering Gynocentric Science." In *Feminism and Science*, edited by N. Tuna. Bloomington: Indiana University Press.

Gordon, Linda, and Allen Hunter. 1977–78. "Sex, Family and the New Right: Anti-feminism as a Political Force." *Radical America* 12:8–25.

Gordon, Paul. 1983. *White Law: Racism in the Police, Courts and Prisons*. London: Pluto Press.

Gough, Ian. 1979. *The Political Economy of the Welfare State*. London: Macmillan.

Gouldner, Alvin. 1970. *The Coming Crisis of Western Sociology*. New York: Avon.

Graham, Patricia. 1987. "Home Birth: Folly or Fulfilment." *The Province*, 22 November.

Gramsci, Antonio. 1971. *Selections from the Prison Notebooks*. London: London and Wishart, 1947.

Grau, Charles. 1982. "Whatever Happened to Politics? A Critique of Marxist Structuralist Accounts of State and Law." In *Marxism and Law*, edited by P. Beirne and R. Quinney. San Francisco: Jossey-Bass.

Greater Vancouver Regional District. 1993. Report of the Birth Centre Working Group for the Greater Vancouver Regional District. Vancouver: GVRD.

Griffin, Kevin. 1988. "Victoria to Consider Nurses as Midwives." *Vancouver Sun*, 25 March.

Growe, Sarah Jane. 1991. *Who Cares? The Crisis in Canadian Nursing*. Toronto: McClelland and Stewart.

Hagan, John. 1984. *The Disreputable Pleasures: Crime and Deviance in Canada*, 2d ed. Toronto: Prentice-Hall.

Haire, Doris. 1981. "Improving the Outcome of Pregnancy through Increased Utilization of Midwives." *Journal of Nurse-Midwifery* 26:5–8.

Hamowy, Ronald. 1984. *Canadian Medicine: A Study in Restricted Entry*. Vancouver: The Fraser Institute.

Hanft, Ruth, and Joseph Eichenholz. 1980. "The Regulation of Health Technology." *Proceedings of the Academy of Political Science* 33:148–9.

Hanley, Fiona. 1993. "Midwife-Friendly Care." *Canadian Nurse* 89:13–16.

Harris, Robert, and David Webb. 1987. *Welfare, Power, and Juvenile Justice.* London: Tavistock.

Harrison, Michelle. 1983. *A Woman in Residence.* Harmondsworth: Penguin.

Hart, Donn V. 1965. "From Pregnancy through Birth in a Bisayan Filipino Village." In *Southeast Asian Birth Customs: Three Studies in Human Reproduction*, edited by D. Hart, P. Rajadhon, and R. Coughlin, 1–113. New Haven, Human Relations Area Files Press.

Hart, Nicky. 1982. "Is Capitalism Bad for Your Health?" *British Journal of Sociology* 33(3): 435–43.

Haug, Marie R., and Bebe Lavin. 1979. "Public Challenge of Physician Authority." *Medical Care* 17(8): 844–58.

Haun, Nancy. 1984. "Nursing Care During Labor." *Canadian Nurse* 80(9): 26–9.

Hazell, Lester. 1974. *Birth Goes Home.* Seattle: Catalyst.

Hedin, Barbara, and Joan Donovan. 1989. "A Feminist Perspective on Nursing Education." *Nurse Educator* 14:8–13.

Hedstrom, Louise, and Niles Newton. 1986. "Touch in Labor: A Comparison of Cultures and Eras." *Birth* 13(3):181–6.

Hefti, Renee. 1992. "Protection, Promotion, and Support: The Health Professional's Role." *British Columbia Medical Journal* 34:95–9.

Held, David. 1983. "Introduction: Central Perspectives on the Modern State." In *States and Societies*, edited by D. Held, J. Anderson, B. Gieben, S. Hall, L. Harris, P. Lewis, N. Parker, and B. Turok. Oxford: Martin Robertson.

Held, David, and Joel Kreiger. 1983. "Accumulation, Legitimation and the State: The Ideas of Claus Offe and Jurgen Habermas." In *States and Societies*, edited by D. Held et al. Oxford: Martin Robertson.

Herbert, Pearl. 1993. "Is Midwifery Education New to Canada?" *Edufacts* (Summer): 3–4.

Hewat, Roberta. 1992. "Preparing Mothers: Prenatal Lactation Assessment." *British Columbia Medical Journal* 34:88–90.

Hicks, C. 1992. "Research in Midwifery: Are Midwives Their Own Worst Enemies?" *Midwifery* 8:12–18.

Hird, Carol, and Brian Burtch. 1991. "Midwifery in Canada." *Japanese Journal for Midwives* 45:48–54.

Hobbes, Thomas. 1974. *Leviathan.* Edited by C.B. Macpherson. Harmondsworth: Penguin (originally published 1651).

Hobel, C.J. 1976. "Recognition of the High Risk Pregnant Woman." In *Management of the High Risk Pregnancy*, edited by W.N. Spellacy. Baltimore: University Park Press.

"Home Birth Percentages." 1992. MIDIRS *Midwifery Digest* 2(3): 310.

Hood, Hugh. 1985. *Reservoir Ravine.* Toronto: General Publishing.

hooks, bell. 1989. *Talking Back: Thinking Feminist, Thinking Black*. Boston: South End Press.

Howitz, Peter, and Jytte Ussing. 1978. "Home or Hospital Deliveries: An Analysis of the Wishes of 5,240 Danish Women Concerning the Place of Delivery." *Ugeskrift For Laeger* 140(26): 1569–73.

Hsia, Lily. 1991. "Midwives and the Empowerment of Women: An International Perspective." *Journal of Nurse-Midwifery* 36(2): 85–7.

Hughes, Everett Cherrington, Helen MacGill Hughes, and Irwin Deutscher. 1958. *Twenty Thousand Nurses Tell Their Story: A Report on Nursing Functions Sponsored by the American Nurses' Association*. Philadelphia: Lippincott.

Hull, V.J. 1979. "Women, Doctors and Family Health Care: Some Lessons from Rural Java." *Studies in Family Planning* 10(11–12): 315–25.

Ignatieff, Michael. 1981. "State, Civil Society, and Total Institutions: A Critique of Recent Social Histories of Punishment." In *Crime and Justice: An Annual Review of Research*, vol. 3, edited by Michael Tonry and Norval Morris. Chicago, University of Chicago Press. Reprinted in S. Cohen and A. Scull, eds., *Social Control and the State*. Oxford: Basil Blackwell 1985.

Illich, Ivan. 1977. *Limits to Medicine*. Harmondsworth: Penguin.

ICEA Board of Directors. 1985. "ICEA Resolution on Midwifery in Canada." Typescript.

– 1989. "ICEA Adopts New Resolutions." *International Journal of Childbirth Education* (May) 5.

International Confederation of Midwives, World Health Organization, and United Nations Children's Fund. 1987. *Women's Health and the Midwife: A Global Perspective*. Geneva: World Health Organization.

International Federation of Gynaecology and Obstetrics and International Confederation of Midwives. 1976. "International Definition of Midwifery." In *Maternity Care in the World*, 2d ed. Oxford: Pergamon Press.

Issalys, Pierre. 1978. "The Professions Tribunal and the Control of Ethical Conduct among Professionals." *McGill Law Journal* 24:588–626.

Jacobson, Doranne. 1974. "The Women of North and Central India: Goddesses and Wives." In *Many Sisters: Women in Cross-Cultural Perspective*, edited by C. Mathiasson. New York: Free Press.

Jacobson, Helga E. 1979. "Women's Perspectives in Research." *Atlantis* 4:98–107.

Jankovic, Ivan. 1980. "Social Class and Criminal Sentencing." In *Punishment and Penal Discipline*, edited by Tony Platt and Paul Takagi. Berkeley: Crime and Justice Associates.

Jeffery, Patricia, Roger Jeffery, and Andrew Lyon. 1989. *Labour Pains and Labour Power: Women and Childbearing in India*. London: Zed Books.

Jensen, Margaret D., Ralph C. Benson, and Irene M. Bobak. 1979. *Maternity Care: The Nurse and the Family*. St. Louis: C.V. Mosby.

Jessop, Bob. 1982. *The Capitalist State*. Oxford: Martin Robertson.

Jiminez, M. 1990. "Midwife Must Stand Trial, Judge Decides." *Globe and Mail*, 10 November.

Jordan, Brigitte. 1980. *Birth in Four Cultures: A Crosscultural Investigation of Childbirth in Yucatan, Holland, Sweden, and the United States*. Montreal: Eden Press.

– 1981. "Studying Childbirth: The Experience and Methods of a Woman Anthropologist." In *Childbirth: Alternatives to Medical Control*, edited by S. Romalis. Austin: University of Texas Press.

– 1987. "High Technology: The Case of Obstetrics." *World Health Forum* 8:312–33.

Kargar, I. 1990. "Traditional Midwifery Skills." *Nursing Times* 86(23): 74–5.

Kaufman, Karen. 1989. "Midwifery on Trial." *The Midwifery Task Force Journal* 2: 1–2 (Ontario).

Kershaw, Anne. 1986. "Save Home-Birth Tradition: Midwife." *Kingston Whig-Standard*, 30 October.

Kinch, Robert A.H. 1986. "Midwifery and Home Births." *Canadian Medical Association Journal* 135(4): 280–1.

Kirby, Sandra, and Kate McKenna. 1989. *Experience, Research, Social Change: Methods for the Margin*. Toronto: Garamond Press.

Kitahara, Ryuju. 1982. "Health Care and Medicine in Japan." Presentation to the Department of Anthropology and Sociology, University of British Columbia, 11 March.

Kitzinger, Jenny. 1990. "Strategies of the Early Childbirth Movement: A Case-Study of the National Childbirth Trust." In *The Politics of Maternity Care: Services for Childbearing Women in Twentieth-Century Britain*, edited by J. Garcia, R. Kilpatrick, and M. Richards. Oxford: Clarendon Press.

Kitzinger, Sheila. 1978. *Women as Mothers*. Glasgow: Fontana.

– 1978a. "Women's Experience of Birth at Home." In *The Place of Birth*, edited by Sheila Kitzinger and John A. Davis. Oxford: Oxford University Press.

– ed. 1988. *The Midwife Challenge*. London: Pandora.

– 1990. "Midwifery in the 90s." Paper presented to Midwives Association of British Columbia, Vancouver, 9 November.

– 1991. *Homebirth: The Essential Guide to Giving Birth Outside of the Hospital*. Toronto: Macmillan.

Kitzinger, Sheila, and John A. Davis, eds. 1978. *The Place of Birth: A Study of the Environment in Which Birth Takes Place with Special Reference to Home Confinements*. Oxford: Oxford University Press.

Klein, Michael C. 1993. Personal communication with author (3 August).

Klein, Michael, I. Lloyd, C. Redman, M. Bull, and A.C. Turnbull. 1993. "A Comparison of Low-Risk Women Booked for Delivery in Two Systems of Care: Shared-Care (Consultant) and Integrated General Practice Unit. I. Obstetrical Procedures and Neonatal Outcome. II. Labour and Delivery Management and Neonatal Outcome." *British Journal of Obstetrics and Gynaecology* 90:118–22 and 123–28.

Klein, Michael, Robert Gauthier, Sally Jorgensen, James Robbins, Janusz Kaczorowski, Barbara Johnson, Marjollaine Corriveau, Ruta Westrelch, Kathy Waghorn, Morrie Gelfand, Melvin Guralnick, Gary Luskey, and Arvind Joshi. 1993. "Episiotomy as a Prevention Strategy: Does It Work?" *Journal of the Society of Obstetricians and Gynecologists of Canada* 15(5): 590–602.

Klein, Sandra. 1980. "A Childbirth Manual," rev. ed. Typescript.

Kloosterman, Gerrit Jan. 1981. "Organization of Obstetric Care in the Netherlands." In *Midwifery is a Labour of Love.* Vancouver: Maternal Health Society.

Knickerbocker, Nancy. 1980. "Genetic Defect: An Early Warning." *Vancouver Sun,* 7 November.

Knutilla, Murray. 1987. *State Theories: From Liberalism to the Challenge of Feminism.* Toronto: Garamond Press.

– 1992. *State Theories,* 2d ed. Halifax: Fernwood.

Korcok, Milan. 1972. "Can the Midwife Find a Home in Canada?" *Medical Post* 8(5), 11.

– 1972a. "Health Planners Debate the Midwife's Role: Her Capabilities Are Unquestioned, but Acceptance Hinges on Physician and Patient Reactions". *Medical Post* 8(4), 7, 45.

Korones, Sheldon, and Jean Lancaster. 1986. *High-Risk Newborn Infants: The Basis for Intensive Nursing Care.* St. Louis: C.V. Mosby.

Kraus, Nancy. 1984. "Cost-Effectiveness at Whose Cost?" *Journal of Nurse-Midwifery* 29:1–2.

Kwast, Barbara. 1991. "Maternal Mortality: The Magnitude and the Causes." *Midwifery* 7(1): 4–7.

– 1993. "Safe Motherhood: The First Decade." Keynote address at the Twenty-third Triennal Congress of the International Confederation of Midwives, Vancouver, 10 May.

Labonte, Ronald. 1983. "Good Health: Individual or Social." *Canadian Forum* (April) 10–13.

Laderman, Carol. 1983. *Wives and Midwives: Childbirth and Nutrition in Rural Malaysia.* Berkeley: University of California Press.

Lang, Dorothea. 1979. "Modern Midwifery." In *Maternal and Infant Care,* edited by Elizabeth Dickason and Martha Schult. New York: McGraw-Hill.

Lang, Raven. 1972. *Birth Book*. Palo Alto: Genesis Press.

Larkin, Gerald. 1983. *Occupational Monopoly and Modern Medicine*. London: Tavistock.

Larsen, E.N. 1992. Personal communication with author (14 May).

Larson, Magali Sarfatti. 1977. *The Rise of Professionalism: A Sociological Analysis*. Berkeley: University of California Press.

Leavitt, Judith. 1980. "Birthing and Anesthesia: The Debate over Twilight Sleep." *Signs: Journal of Women in Culture and Society* 6:147–64.

Lee, Lois. 1972. "Pregnancy and Childbirth Practices of the Northern Roglai." *Southeast Asia* 2(1): 26–52.

Lessing, Doris. 1986. "Prisons We Choose to Live In." *Canadian Forum* (February) 10–17.

Letty, Carol-Anne. 1993. Birth Statistics 1 July 1992 to 30 June 1993. Typescript.

Levy, Barry, Frederick Wilkinson, and William Marine. 1971. "Reducing Neonatal Mortality Rate with Nurse-Midwives." *American Journal of Obstetrics and Gynecology* 109:50–8.

Lewis, Paul. 1991. "Men in Midwifery: Their Experiences as Students and as Practitioners." In *Midwives, Research and Childbirth*, vol. 2, edited by Sarah Robinson and Ann Thomson. London: Chapman and Hall.

Light, Linda. 1981. "Feminism and Collectivity: The Integrative Function." MA thesis, University of British Columbia.

Lim, Linda Y.C. 1983. "Capitalism, Imperialism, and Patriarchy: The Dilemma of Third-World Women Workers in Multinational Factories." In *Women, Men, and the International Division of Labor*, edited by J. Nash and M. Fernandez-Kelly. Albany: State University of New York Press.

Lin, Nan. 1976. *Methods of Social Research*. Toronto: McGraw-Hill.

Lithell, Ulla-Britt. 1981. "Breast-feeding Habits and Their Relation to Infant Mortality and Marital Fertility." *Journal of Family History* 6:182–94.

Lipset, Seymour Martin. 1986. "Historical Traditions and National Characteristics: A Comparative Analysis of Canada and the United States." *Canadian Journal of Sociology* 11:113–56.

Litoff, Judy. 1978. *American Midwives: 1860 to the Present*. Westport, Conn.: Riverside Press.

Little, Ruth E., and Ann Pytkowicz. 1978. "Drinking during Pregnancy in Alcoholic Women." *Alcoholism* 2:179–83.

Lorber, Judith. 1975. "Women and Medical Sociology: Invisible Professionals and Ubiquitous Patients." In *Another Voice: Feminist Perspectives on Social Life and Social Science*, edited by Marcia Hillman and Rosabeth Kanter. Garden City, Anchor Books.

Lugrin, N. de Bertrand. 1928. *The Pioneer Women of Vancouver Island, 1843–1866*. Victoria: Women's Canadian Club of Victoria.

Lubic, Ruth W. 1981. "Alternative Maternity Care: Resistance and Change." In *Childbirth: Alternatives to Medical Control*, edited by S. Romalis. Austin: University of Texas Press.

– 1983. "Child Birthing Centers: Delivering More for Less." *American Journal of Nursing* 83:1053–6.

– 1992. "The Alternative or the Norm for the Future?" *Australian College of Midwives Journal* 3:6–14.

McClain, Carol. 1975. "Ethno-obstetrics in Ajijic." *Anthropological Quarterly* 48:38–56.

McClung, Nellie. 1935. *Clearing in the West*. Toronto: Thomas Allen.

McIntosh, J. 1989. "Models of Childbirth and Social Class: A Study of 80 Working-Class Primigravidae." In *Midwives, Research and Childbirth*, vol. 1, edited by Sarah Robinson and Ann Thomson. London: Chapman and Hall.

McIntyre, Greg. 1983. "Midwives Ask for Sanction of Law." *The Province*, 18 February.

MacIntyre, Sally. 1979. "Some Issues in the Study of Pregnancy Careers". *Sociological Review* 27(4): 755–71.

MacIsaac, Ronald. 1976. "Negligence Actions against Medical Doctors." *Chitty's Law Journal* 24:201–6.

McKinlay, J., and S. McKinlay. 1976. "The Questionable Contribution of Medical Measures to the Decline of Mortality in the United States in the Twentieth Century." *Millbank Memorial Fund Quarterly* 55:405–28.

McLaren, Angus, and Arlene McLaren. 1986. *The Bedroom and the State: The Changing Practices and Politics of Contraception and Abortion in Canada, 1880–1980*. Toronto: McClelland and Stewart.

McMillan, Carol. 1982. *Women, Reason and Nature*. Princeton: Princeton University Press.

McMullan, John, and R.S. Ratner. 1983. "State, Labour, and Justice in British Columbia." In *Deviant Designations*, edited by T. Fleming and L. Visano. Toronto: Butterworths.

McRae, Kenneth. 1979. "The Plural Society and the Western Political Tradition." *Canadian Journal of Political Science* 12:675–89.

Maine, Deborah. 1986. "Maternal Mortality: Helping Women Off the Road to Death." *WHO Chronicle* 40(5): 175–83.

– n.d. *Safe Motherhood Programs: Options and Issues*. New York: Center for Population and Family Health (Columbia University).

Mandel, Michael. 1987. "'Relative Autonomy' and the Criminal Justice Apparatus." In *Criminal Justice Politics in Canada*, edited by R.S. Ratner and J.L. McMullan. Vancouver: University of British Columbia Press.

– 1989. *The Charter of Rights and the Legalization of Politics in Canada*. Toronto: Wall and Thompson Inc.

Mani, S.B. 1980. "A Review of Midwife Training Programs in Tamil-Nadju." *Studies in Family Planning* 11:395–400.

Manitoba. Office of the Chief Medical Examiner. 1992. *Annual Report 1990*. Winnipeg: Department of Justice.

Mankoff, Milton. 1970. "Power in Advanced Capitalist Society: A Review Essay on Recent Elitist and Marxist Criticisms of Pluralist Theory." *Social Problems* 17:418–30.

Marieskind, Helen I. 1980. *Women in the Health System: Patients, Providers, and Programs*. Toronto: C.V. Mosby.

Martin, Emily. 1987. *The Woman in the Body: A Cultural Analysis of Reproduction*. Boston: Beacon Press.

Marx, Karl, and Friedrich Engels. 1979. *The Communist Manifesto*. Harmondsworth: Penguin (originally published in 1872).

Mason, Jutta. 1988. "Midwifery in Canada." In *The Midwife Challenge*, edited by S. Kitzinger. London: Pandora.

– 1987. "A History of Midwifery in Canada." In *Report of the Task Force on the Implementation of Midwifery in Ontario*, appendix 1. Toronto: Province of Ontario.

Matthews, J.S. 1947. "Letter re: Fred H. Goodrich's 'Victorian Order Born in Vancouver.'" *Daily Province* 10 November (letter dated 17 November 1947); file folder 17: "Victorian Order of Nurses," Vancouver City Archives.

– 1945. "Mid-wives." Typescript. File folder 175, Vancouver City Archives.

Maynard, Eileen. 1974. "Guatemalan Women: Life under Two Types of Patriarchy." In *Many Sisters: Women in Cross-Cultural Perspective*, edited by C. Mathiasson. New York: Free Press.

Meenan, A., I. Gaskin, P. Hunt, and C. Ball. 1992. "A New (Old) Maneuver for the Management of Shoulder Dystocia." MIDIRS *Midwifery Digest* 2:306–10.

Mehl, Louis. 1977. "Outcomes of Elective Home Births: A Series of 1,146 Cases." *Journal of Reproductive Medicine* 19:281–90.

Melucci, Antonio. 1988. "New Perspectives on Social Movements: An Interview with Alberto Melucci." In *Nomads of the Past and Present: Social Movements and Individual Needs in Contemporary Society*, edited by J. Keane and P. Mier. London: Radius.

Menzies, Ken. 1982. *Sociological Theory in Use*. London: Routledge and Kegan Paul.

Midelfort, H.C. Eric. 1972. *Witch Hunting in South Western Germany: The Social and Intellectual Foundations*. Stanford: Stanford University Press.

Midwifery and the Law. 1991. Videotape produced by the Department of Continuing Studies, Simon Fraser University, and the Knowledge Network of British Columbia.

Midwives Association of British Columbia. 1984. "Guidelines to Midwifery Practice." Vancouver: MABC.

– 1993. Presentation to the Health Professions Council, Vancouver, 25 January.

Miliband, Ralph. 1972. "The Problem of the Capitalist State: Reply to Nicos Poulantzas." In *Ideology in Social Science*, edited by R. Blackburn. London: Fontana/Collins.

– 1973. *The State in Capitalist Society*. London: Quartet.

Millman, Marcia. 1978. *The Unkindest Cut: Life in the Backrooms of Medicine*. New York: William Morrow.

Mills, C.W. 1959. *The Sociological Imagination*. Oxford: Oxford University Press.

Mills, Donald, and Donald Larsen. 1986. "The Professionalization of Canadian Chiropractic." In *Health and Canadian Society: Sociological Perspectives*, edited by D. Coburn, C. D'Arcy, P. New, and G. Torrance. Toronto: Fitzhenry and Whiteside.

Minchin, Maureen. 1985. *Breastfeeding Matters: What We Need to Know about Infant Feeding*. Alfredton, Victoria, N.S.W.: Alma Publications and George Allen & Unwin.

Mitchinson, Wendy. 1979. "Historical Attitudes toward Women and Childbirth." *Atlantis* 4: 13–34.

– 1991. *The Nature of Their Bodies: Women and Their Doctors in Victorian Canada*. Toronto: University of Toronto Press.

Mitford, Jessica. 1992. *The American Way of Birth*. New York: Penguin Books.

Mittelbach, Margaret. 1986. "The Midwife Crisis." *Los Angeles Free Weekly*, 12 December.

Morton, Desmond (with Terry Copp). 1980. *Working People*. Ottawa: Deneau and Greenberg.

Morton, F.L. 1993. *Morgentaler v. Borowski: Abortion, the Charter, and the Courts*. Toronto: McClelland and Stewart.

Mouzelis, Nicos. 1984. "On the Crisis of Marxist Theory." *British Journal of Criminology* 35: 112–21.

Movimiento Pro Parto Humanizado (Movement for Humanitarian Birth). 1993. "Derechos Fundamentales de la Mujer Embarazada (Fundamental Rights of the Pregnant Woman)." Poster from Uruguay, displayed at 1993 ICM Congress, Vancouver.

Moysa, Marilyn, and Sherri Aikenhead. 1991. "Judge Finds Midwife Not Guilty of Illegally Practising Medicine." *Edmonton Journal*, 6 June.

Muzio, Lois. 1991. "Midwifery Education and Nursing: Curricular Education or Civil War?" *Nursing and Health Care* 12:376–79.

Myles, Margaret. 1975. *Textbook for Midwives*, 10th ed. London: Churchill Livingstone.

Nagy, Doreen. 1983–84. "Obstetrical Forceps: Symbols of Power and Professionalism in Victorian Britain." *Nexus* 31:98–103.

Navarro, Vicente. 1976. *Medicine under Capitalism*. New York: Prodist.

– 1976a. "The Political and Economic Determinants of Health and Health Care in Rural America." *Inquiry* 13:111–21.

– 1986. *Crisis, Health, and Medicine: A Social Critique*. London: Tavistock.

Nasah, B.T. 1991. "Midwives: The Key to Safe Motherhood." *World Health Forum* 12: 7–9.

Naylor, C.D. 1981. "A Feeling of Déjà Vu: The CMA and Health Insurance." *This Magazine* (July–August) 9–14.

Neilans, Mary. 1992. "Midwifery: From Recognition to Regulation – The Perils of Government Intervention." *Healthsharing* (Summer–Fall) 27–9.

Nelson, M. 1983. "Working-Class Women, Middle-Class Women, and Models of Childbirth." *Social Problems* 30(3): 284–97.

New York Academy of Medicine. 1933. *Maternal Mortality in New York City: A Study of all Puerperal Deaths in 1930–1932*. New York: Commonwealth Fund.

Noble, Elizabeth. 1983. *Childbirth with Insight*. Boston: Houghton Mifflin.

Oakley, Ann. 1976. "Wisewoman and Medicine Man: Changes in the Management of Childbirth." In *The Rights and Wrongs of Women*, edited by J. Mitchell and A. Oakley. Harmondsworth: Penguin.

– 1980. *Women Confined: Towards a Sociology of Childbirth*. New York: Schocken Books.

– 1984. *The Captured Womb: A History of Medical Care of Women*. London: Basil Blackwell.

O'Brien, Mary. 1981. *The Politics of Reproduction*. London: Routledge and Kegan Paul.

O'Connor, John. 1973. *The Fiscal Crisis of the State*. New York: St. Martin's Press.

Odent, Michael. 1981. "The Evolution of Obstetrics at Pithiviers." *Birth and the Family Journal* 8:7–15.

– 1986. *Primal Health: A Blueprint for Our Survival*. London: Century Hutchinson.

Ohnuki-Tierney, Emiko. 1984. *Illness and Culture in Contemporary Japan*. Cambridge: Cambridge University Press.

Olsen, Dennis. 1980. *The State Elite*. Toronto: McClelland and Stewart.

O'Neill, John. 1986. "The Medicalization of Social Control." *Canadian Review of Sociology and Anthropology* 23(3): 350–64.

Ontario. 1987. *Report of the Task Force on the Implementation of Midwifery in Ontario*. Toronto: Province of Ontario.

Ontario Association of Midwives and the Nurse Midwives Association of Ontario. 1983. "Brief on Midwifery Care in Ontario." Brief submitted to the Health Disciplines Review Committee, Toronto (December).

Ontario Interim Regulatory Council on Midwifery. 1991. "Aboriginal
    Women's Group Adopts Resolution on Midwifery Profession." *The Gazette*
    2:3.

– 1992. "Federation of University Women Adopts Resolution on Mid-
    wifery." *The Gazette* 3:4.

Osborne, Judith. 1983. "The Prosecutor's Discretion to Withdraw Criminal
    Cases in the Lower Courts." *Canadian Journal of Criminology* 25:55–78.

Padmore, Tim. 1983. "Vancouver Hospital Tries Midwifery Program." *(Mon-
    treal) Gazette*, 21 February.

Page, Lesley. 1993. "Midwives Hear the Heartbeat of the Future." In *Pro-
    ceedings of the Twenty-third Triennial Congress of the International Confedera-
    tion of Midwives*, vol. 3, 1477–88. Vancouver: Midwives Association of
    British Columbia.

Paine, Lisa. 1991. "Midwifery Education and Research in the Future."
    Journal of Nurse-Midwifery 36(3): 199–203.

Panitch, Leo. 1979. "The Role and Nature of the Canadian State." In *The
    Canadian State: Political Economy and Political Power*, edited by L. Panitch.
    Toronto: University of Toronto Press.

Paul, Alexandra. 1990. "Stillbirth Prompts New Pressure to Legalize Mid-
    wifery." *Winnipeg Free Press*, 10 May.

Pearse, Warren. 1977. "Home Birth Crisis." ACOG *Newsletter*.

– 1979. "Home Birth: Editorial." *Journal of the American Medical Association*
    241: 1039–41.

Pelletier, Gertrude. 1988. "Avis favorable aux sages-femmes." *The Canadian
    Nurse/L'infirmière Canadienne* 84:43.

Peng, J.Y. et al. 1972. "Village Midwives in Malaysia." *Studies in Family
    Planning* 3:25–8.

Phaff, J.M.L., L. Sassi, L. Valvanne, and E.J. Hickl. 1975. *Midwives
    in Europe: Present and Future Education and Role of the Midwife in Coun-
    cil of Europe Member States and in Finland.* Strasbourg: Council of
    Europe.

Phillips, Paul, and Erin Phillips. 1983. *Women and Work: Inequality in the
    Labour Market.* Toronto: James Lorimer.

Picard, André. 1991. "Midwives No Longer Shrugging Off Attacks." *Globe
    and Mail*, 29 November.

Placek, Paul, and Selma Taffel. 1980. "Trends in Cesarean Section Rates for
    the United States, 1970–1978." *Public Health Reports* 95:540–1.

Plommer, Leslie. 1979. "Male Midwives Meet Opposition in Britain." *Globe
    and Mail*, 15 February.

Poulantzas, Nicos. 1972. "The Problem of the Capitalist State." In *Ideology in
    Social Science*, edited by R. Blackburn. London: Fontana.

– 1978. *Political Power and Social Classes.* London: New Left Books.

– 1980. *State, Power, Socialism.* London: New Left Books.

Raphael, Dana. 1975. "Matresence, Becoming a Mother, a 'New/Old' Rite de Passage." In *Being Female*, edited by D. Raphael. The Hague: Mouton.

Rasmussen, Linda, Lorna Rasmussen, Candace Savage, and Anne Wheeler. 1976. *A Harvest Yet to Reap: A History of Prairie Women*. Toronto: The Women's Press.

Ratner, R.S., John McMullan, and Brian Burtch. 1987. "The Problem of Relative Autonomy and Criminal Justice in the Canadian State." In *State Control: Criminal Justice Politics in Canada*, edited by R.S. Ratner and J.L. McMullan. Vancouver: University of British Columbia Press.

Ray, Barb. 1988. "Letter to the Editor." *Victoria Times-Colonist* (May).

Reasons, Charles, and Duncan Chappell. 1985. "Crooked Lawyers: Towards a Political Economy of Deviance in the Profession." In *The New Criminologies in Canada: State, Crime, and Control*, edited by T. Fleming. Toronto: Oxford University Press.

Registered Nurses Association of British Columbia. 1979. "RNABC Moves on Midwifery." *RNABC News* 11(5): 20–3.

– 1987. "Position Statement: Midwifery." *RNABC News* (July–August).

Reid, Anthony, and J. Grant Galbraith. 1988. "Midwifery in a Family Practice: A Pilot Study." *Canadian Family Physician* 34: 1887–90.

Relyea, Joyce. 1992. "The Rebirth of Midwifery in Canada: An Historical Perspective." *Midwifery* 8(4): 159.

Renaud, Marc. 1978. "On the Structural Constraints to State Intervention in Health." In *The Cultural Crisis of Modern Medicine*, edited by J. Ehrenreich. New York: Monthly Review Press.

Renzetti, Claire, and Daniel Curran. 1989. *Women, Men, and Society: The Sociology of Gender*. Boston: Allyn and Bacon.

Report of the Director-General. 1991. *Child Health and Development: Health of the Newborn*. Geneva: World Health Organization.

Riddell, David. 1992. "The Uniqueness of Human Milk." *British Columbia Medical Journal* 34:85–7.

Riessman, Catherine Kohler. 1992. "Women and Medicalization: A New Perspective." In *Perspectives in Medical Sociology*, edited by Phil Brown. Prospect Heights, Ill.: Waveland Press.

Rifkin, Susan. 1990. *Community Participation in Maternal and Child Health/ Family Planning Programmes*. Geneva: World Health Organization.

Robertson, Ann. 1990. "Letter to the Editor." *RNABC News* 22:5.

Robinson, Sarah and Ann Thompson, eds. 1991. *Midwives, Research and Childbirth*, vol. 2. London: Chapman and Hill.

Romalis, Shelly, ed. 1981. *Childbirth: Alternatives to Medical Control*. Austin: University of Texas Press.

Rooks, Judith, and Susan Fischman. 1980. "American Nurse-Midwifery Practice in 1976–1977: Reflections on 50 Years of Growth and Development." *American Journal of Public Health* 70:990–6.

Rose, Barbara Wade. 1992. "Delivering a Message about Childbirth." *Globe and Mail*, 23 December.

Rosenau, Pauline. 1992. *Postmodernism and the Social Sciences*. Princeton: Princeton University Press.

Rossi, Alice. 1976. *The Feminist Papers: From Beauvoir to Adams*. New York: Bantam.

Rothman, Barbara Katz. 1983. "Anatomy of a Compromise: Nurse-Midwifery and the Rise of the Birth Center." *Journal of Nurse-Midwifery* 28:3–7.

– 1984. *Giving Birth: Alternatives in Childbirth*. Harmondsworth: Penguin.

Rowbotham, Sheila. 1973. *Hidden From History*. London: Pluto Press.

Royston, Erica, and Sue Armstrong, eds. 1989. *Preventing Maternal Deaths*. Geneva: World Health Organization.

Ruzek, Sheryl. 1991. "Feminist Visions of Health: An International Perspective." In *Perspectives in Medical Sociology*, edited by Phil Brown. Prospect Heights, Ill.: Waveland Press.

Sallomi, Pacia, Angie Pallow, and Peggy O'Mara McMahon. 1981. "Midwifery and the Law." *Mothering* 21:63–83.

Salvage, Wendy. 1986. *The Politics of Nursing*. London: Heinemann Nursing.

Samuels, Alec. 1974. "Injuries to Unborn Children." *Alberta Law Review* 12:266–70.

Schreier, A. 1983. "The Tucson Nurse-Midwifery Service: The First Four Years." *Journal of Nurse-Midwifery* 28:24–30.

Schroeder, Andreas. 1980. "Birthright." *Today Magazine*, 4 October.

Scully, Diana. 1980. *Men Who Control Women's Health: The Miseducation of Obstetrician-Gynecologists*. Boston: Houghton Mifflin.

Scupholme, Anne. 1982. "Nurse-Midwives and Physicians: A Team Approach to Obstetrical Care in a Perinatal Center." *Journal of Nurse-Midwifery* 27:21–7.

Seager, Joni, and Ann Olson. 1986. *Women in the World: An International Atlas*. London: Pan Books.

Shea, Lois. 1991. "To Moscow, with Love: Carol Leonard Is Horrified – but Hopeful – about Conditions in Moscow's Birth Houses." *Concord Monitor*, 24 January.

Shenker, Lewis, R. Post, and J. Seiler. 1975. "Routine Electronic Monitoring of Fetal Heart Rate and Uterine Activity during Labor." *Obstetrics and Gynecology* 46:185–9.

Shoalts, David. 1991. "Ontario Recognizes Midwifery." *Globe and Mail*, 22 November.

Shorter, Edward. 1982. *A History of Women's Bodies*. Toronto: University of Toronto Press.

Shortt, S.E.D. 1981. "Antiquarians and Amateurs: Reflections on the Writing of Medical History in Canada." In *Medicine in Canadian Society:*

Historical Perspectives, edited by S. Shortt. Montreal: McGill-Queen's University Press.

– 1983–4. "The Hospital in the Nineteenth Century." *Journal of Canadian Studies* 18:3–14.

Sidel, Ruth. 1973. *Women and Child Care in China*. Baltimore: Penguin.

Sigerist, Henry. 1944. *Saskatchewan Health Services Survey Commission: Report of the Commissioner*. Regina: King's Printer.

Sinquefield, Gail. 1983. "A Malpractice Dilemma: Defining Standards of Care for Certified Nurse-Midwives." *Journal of Nurse-Midwifery* 28:1–2.

Smart, Carol. 1989. *Feminism and the Power of Law*. London: Routledge and Kegan Paul.

Smith, Elizabeth. 1980. *A Woman with a Purpose*. Toronto: University of Toronto Press.

Smith, Marcia. 1976. "Changing Health Hazards in Infancy and Childhood in Northern Canada." In *Circumpolar Health*, edited by Roy J. Shephard and S. Itoh. Toronto: University of Toronto Press.

Smith, W. Eugene. 1951. "Nurse Midwife: Maude Callen Eases Pain of Birth, Life and Death." *Life* 31: 134–45.

Smith-Bowen, E. 1964. *Return to Laughter: An Anthropological Novel*. New York: Doubleday.

Society of Obstetricians and Gynecologists of Canada. 1986. "SOGC Statement on Midwifery Approved at the Annual Business Meeting." Typescript.

Sorley, Jane Hamilton. 1851–93. "Records of Births attended in Five Islands-Economy Area [Nova Scotia], 1851–1893." Mount Allison University Archives, Sackville, Nova Scotia.

Spastics Society. 1981. "A Charter for the Eighties." Joint statement on maternity and neonatal services supported by fourteen voluntary and professional groups (May).

Spitzer, Steven. 1983. "Marxist Perspectives in the Sociology of Law." *Annual Review of Sociology* 9: 103–24.

Stanko, Elizabeth. 1990. *Everyday Violence: How Women and Men Experience Sexual and Physical Danger*. London: Pandora Books.

Stanworth, Michelle, ed. 1987. *Reproductive Technologies: Gender, Motherhood, and Medicine*. Oxford: Basil Blackwell.

Starr, Paul. 1978. "Medicine and the Waning of Professional Sovereignty." *Daedalus* 107: 175–93.

– 1980. "Changing the Balance of Power in American Medicine." *The Millbank Memorial Fund Quarterly: Health and Society* 58: 166–72.

– 1983. *The Social Transformation of American Medicine*. New York: Basic Books.

Statistics Canada. 1984. (November) *Surgical Procedures and Treatments, 1979–1981*. Ottawa: Supply and Services Canada.

– 1986. *Births and Deaths: Volume I (1984)*. Ottawa: Supply and Services Canada.

– 1992. *Surgical Procedures and Treatments 1989–90*. Ottawa: Supply and Services Canada (catalogue 82-003S2).

Stein, Peter, and John Shand. 1974. *Legal Values in Western Society*. Edinburgh: Edinburgh University Press.

Stephens, Robert. 1984. "Ontario Midwives Merit Legal Status, NDPer Says." *Globe and Mail,* 16 March.

Stewart, Richard, and Linda Clark. 1982. "Nurse-Midwifery Practice in an All-Hospital Birthing Center: 2,050 Births." *Journal of Nurse-Midwifery* 27: 21–6.

Stonier, J., and Monic Beauchemin. 1993. Private memorandum to ICM President (January).

Strong-Boag, Veronica. 1979. "Canada's Women Doctors: Feminism Constrained." In *A Not Unreasonable Claim: Women and Reform in Canada, 1880s–1920s,* edited by Linda Kealey. Toronto: The Women's Press.

– 1988. *The New Day Recalled: Lives of Girls and Women in English Canada, 1919–1939*. Toronto: Copp Clark Pitman.

Student Nurses Association of Illinois. 1979. "Episiotomy as an American Phenomenon." *Journal of Nurse-Midwifery* 24:31.

Sufrin-Dusler, Caroline. 1990. "Vaginal Birth after Caesarean." *ICEA Review* 14(3): 21–32.

Sugarman, Muriel. 1979. "Regionalization of Maternity and Newborn Care: Facts, Fantasies, Flaws, and Fallacies." In *Compulsory Hospitalization or Freedom of Choice in Childbirth,* edited by D. Stewart and L. Stewart. Marble Hill, Mo.: NAPSAC.

Sullivan, Deborah, and Rose Weitz. 1988. *Labor Pains: Modern Midwives and Home Birth*. New Haven: Yale University Press.

Sullivan-LeMay Legal Action Fund. 1988. Flyer (typescript, mimeo).

Sumner, Colin. 1981. "The Rule of Law and Civil Rights in Contemporary Marxist Theory." *Kapitalistate* 9: 63–91.

Sumner, William Graham. 1960. *Folkways*. New York: New American Library.

Sutley, Joyce. 1982. "Montana Midwife." *Mothering* 24: 80–1.

Swartz, Donald. 1979. "The Politics of Reform: Conflict and Accomodation in Canadian Health Policy." In *The Canadian State,* edited by Leo Panitch. Toronto: University of Toronto Press.

Swedlo, Mavis. 1979. "Childbirth at Home." *Canadian Journal of Public Health* 70:307–9.

Sweet, Lois. 1985. "Midwives Are Battling for Their Freedom." *Toronto Star,* 8 April.

Taffel, S., P. Placeck, and C. Kosary. 1992. "Caesarean Section Rates in 1990: An Update." *Birth* 19:21–2.

Taylor, Ian. 1980. "The Law and Order Issue in the British General Election and Canadian Federal Election of 1979: Crime, Populism and the State." *Canadian Journal of Sociology* 5:285–311.

Tew, Marjorie. 1985. "Place of Birth and Perinatal Mortality." *Journal of the Royal College of General Practitioners* 35:390–4.

– 1986. "The Practices of Birth Attendants and the Safety of Birth." *Midwifery* 2: 3–10.

– 1990. *Safer Childbirth? A Critical History of Maternity Care.* London: Chapman and Hall.

Thacker, Stephen B., and H. David Banta. 1983. "Benefits and Risks of Episiotomy: An Interpretative Review of the English Language Literature, 1860–1980." *Obstetrical and Gynecological Survey* 38:322–38.

Thompson, E.P. 1977. *Whigs and Hunters: The Origin of the Black Act.* Harmondsworth: Penguin.

– 1978. *The Poverty of Theory and Other Essays.* London: Merlin.

– 1983. "The Secret State." In *States and Societies*, edited by David Held et al. Oxford: Martin Robertson.

Thompson, Paul. 1978. *The Voice of the Past: Oral History.* Oxford: Oxford University Press.

Thunhurst, Colin. 1982. *It Makes You Sick: The Politics of the NHS.* London: Pluto Press.

Tonkin, Roger. 1981. *Child Health Profile: Birth Events and Infant Outcomes.* Vancouver: Hemlock Printers.

Treichler, Paula. 1990. "Feminism, Medicine, and the Meaning of Childbirth." In *Body/Politics and the Discourses of Justice*, edited by Mary Jacobus, Evelyn F. Keller, and Sally Shuttleworth. London: Routledge, Chapman, and Hall.

Tuna, Nancy, ed. 1989. *Feminism and Science.* Bloomington: Indiana University Press.

Turk, Austin. 1980. "Analyzing Official Deviance: For Nonpartisan Conflict Analyses in Criminology." In *Radical Criminology: The Coming Crises*, edited by James Inciardi. Beverly Hills: Sage.

Twaddle, Andrew. 1982. "From Medical Sociology to the Sociology of Health: Some Changing Concerns in the Sociological Study of Sickness and Treatment." In *Sociology: The State of the Art*, edited by Tom Bottomore et al. London: Sage.

Tyson, Holliday. 1984. "Village Midwifery in Northern India: The Role of the Dai." *Issue* 5:5–6.

– 1989. "A Retrospective Descriptive Study of 1,001 Home Births Attended by Midwives in Toronto between 1983 and 1988." MSc thesis, McMaster University.

Ursel, Jane. 1988. "The State and the Maintenance of Patriarchy: A Case Study of Family, Labour, and Welfare Legislation in Canada." In *Gender and Society: Creating a Canadian Women's Sociology*, edited by Arlene McLaren. Toronto: Copp Clark Pitman.

Van Wagner, Vicki. 1984. "The Current Politics of Midwifery in Ontario." Paper presented at the annual meeting of the Canadian Sociology and Anthropology Association, Guelph, Ontario.

– 1991. "With Women: Community Midwifery in Ontario." M.A. thesis, York University.

Varney, Helen. 1983. *Nurse-Midwifery.* London: Blackwell Scientific Publications.

Ventre, Fran, and Carol Leonard. 1982. "The Future of Midwifery – An Alliance." *Journal of Nurse-Midwifery* 27:23–4.

Velimirovic, Helga, and Boris Velimirovic. 1981. "The Role of Traditional Birth Attendants in Health Services." *Medical Anthropology* 5: 89–106.

Vincent, Andrew. 1987. *Theories of the State.* Oxford: Basil Blackwell.

Wagner, David. 1980. "The Proleterianization of Nursing in the United States." *International Journal of Health Services* 10:271–90.

Wagner, Marsden. 1985. *Having a Baby in Europe.* Copenhagen: World Health Organization.

– 1990. "Appropriate Technology for Birth." *New Zealand College of Midwives Journal* (November) 10–11, 14–15.

Waitzkin, Howard. 1979. "A Marxian Interpretation of the Growth and Development of Coronary Care Technology." *American Journal of Public Health* 69:1260–72.

– 1983. *The Second Sickness: Contradictions of Capitalist Health Care.* New York: Free Press.

Walker, Noreen, Sandy Pullen, and Marilyn Shinyei. 1986. "Birth Stats: Domiciliary Midwifery Report." *Safe Alternatives in Childbirth* (Edmonton, Alberta) 3:5.

Walzer, Michael. 1983. *Spheres of Justice: A Defense of Pluralism and Equality.* New York: Basic Books.

Ward, W. Peter. 1984. *The Mysteries of Montreal: Memoirs of a Midwife.* Vancouver: University of British Columbia Press.

Wayling, Mrs. F.A. Record of births attended, 1916–1918. File R-E422, Saskatchewan Archives Board.

Weaver, Sally. 1972. *Medicine and Politics Among the Grand River Iroquois: A Study of Neo-Conservatives.* Ottawa: National Museum of Man.

Wetherston, Lesley, E. Carty, A. Rice, and D. Tier. 1985. "Hospital-Based Midwifery: Meeting the Needs of Childbearing Women." *Canadian Nurse* 81:35–7.

Whig-Standard News Services. 1986. "Toronto Hospital Makes Bid to Clinically Train Midwives." *Kingston Whig-Standard*, 9 October.

White, Gregory. 1977. "A Comparison of Home and Hospital Delivery Based on 25 Years' Experience with Both." *Journal of Reproductive Medicine* 19(5): 291–2.

Whiting, Beatrice, and John Whiting. 1979. *Children of Six Cultures: A Psycho-Cultural Analysis.* Cambridge: Harvard University Press.

Whitton, Charlotte. 1945. "v.o.n. Stands for Victorious Over Need." *Saturday Night*, 2 June.

Wiecek, Paul. 1990. "Baby's Death Brings Call to Legalize Midwifery." *Winnipeg Free Press*, 25 April.

Williams, Lynne Sears. "Relations between Alberta Midwives, MDS Appear to Be Thawing Despite High-Profile Trial." *Canadian Medical Association Journal* 145(5): 497–8.

Williams, Marne. 1993. "McMaster, Laurentian and Ryerson Get Midwives." *Brock Press*, 6 January.

Williams, Selma, and Pamela Adelman. 1992. *Riding the Nightmare: Women and Witchcraft from the Old World to Colonial Salem.* New York: Harper Perennial.

Wilson, Susan. 1986. *Women, the Family, and the Economy*, 2d ed. Toronto: Prentice-Hall.

Women's Legal Education and Action Fund (LEAF). 1991. "Factum of the Intervener." Filed in the Supreme Court of Canada in *R. v. Sullivan* (1991). Typescript.

Women's Work Project of the Union for Radical Political Economists. 1976. "USA – Women Health Workers." *Women and Health* 1:14–23.

Woodcock, George. 1990. "Five-Year Fascism." *Canadian Forum* (December) 16–18.

Workers' Compensation Board of British Columbia. 1987. *The 16th Annual Report of the Criminal Injury Compensation Act of British Columbia, January 1, 1987–December 31, 1987.* Richmond: Workers' Compensation Board of British Columbia.

World Health Organization. 1987. "Recommendations from the World Health Organization." Reprinted in *California Association of Midwives Letter* (Summer) 9.

Yankauer, Alfred. 1979. "Infant Mortality and Morbidity in the International Year of the Child." *American Journal of Public Health* 69:852–6.

Young, Iris. 1990. *Justice and the Politics of Difference.* Princeton: Princeton University Press.

Yusuf, Ya'qub ibn. 1984. "Learning from Birth – An Interview with Midwife Darlene Birch." *Chautauqua Review* 2:13–23.

Zinn, Howard. 1970. *The Politics of History.* Boston: Beacon Press.

Index

screening of clients 100,
105; complications 126–
7; smoking 111–12
Scully, Diana 140
Scupholme, Anne 19, 140
Seager, Joni 6,86
Shea, Lois 92
Shenker, Lewis 17
shift work 31
Shorter, Edward 70
Shortt, Sam 72–3, 79
shoulder dystocia 92, 171
Sidel, Ruth 93
Sigerist, Henry 14, 79
Sinquefield, Gail 150, 178
Smart, Carol 22, 37–8, 189
Smith, Elizabeth 76
Smith, Marcia 86
Smith, W. Eugene 80–1
Smith-Bowen, E. 87
snowball sampling 24–5
social class: clients 198–9,
202; and health 22; phy-
sician attendance 80;
resistance 45–6, 50;
social history 72; and
state 39, 43
social movements 39, 46,
50. See also midwifery
movement; postmod-
ernism
Society of Obstetricians
and Gynecologists of
Canada (SOGC) 109,
209–10
solidary aid 64–5. See also
community of women;
feminine networks
Sorley, Jane Hamilton
72
Spastics Society 119
spiritual midwifery 89,
136, 186, 197, 213. See
also community mid-
wifery; The Farm;
granny midwives
Spitzer, Steven 52
"splendid ritual" of birth
209
spouses 57–8

state: and civil society 48–
9; containing struggles
12, 17, 21; "cult of leadership" 40; definitions
of 42–3, 49; enabling
powers 23, 37; "factor of
cohesion" 43; and ideo-
logical structures 14;
suppressing midwifery
17
state theories: conserva-
tism 26, 38–41; cultur-
alism 52; instrumental-
ism 14–15, 24, 47, 52,
61; liberal-pluralism 21,
26; Marxism 42–3; neo-
Marxism 14, 26, 47;
structuralism 14, 21, 23,
39, 43–4, 46, 52, 60–1,
and health 49; modified
224
statism 13–14, 45, 47, 214
Stanko, Elizabeth 207
Starr, Paul 18, 61, 80–1,
142
Statistics Canada 106, 114,
118, 121, 195
Stein, Peter 212
Stephens, Robert 57
Stewart, Richard 19
stillbirths 118, 123, 125,
128–9, 132–3
Stonier, J. 138
Strong-Boag, Veronica 16,
72, 74, 76, 79
Student Nurses Associa-
tion of Illinois, 17
suctioning 122, 124
Sufrin-Dusler, Caroline
164
Sugarman, Muriel 143
Sullivan, Deborah 82–3
Sullivan-LeMay (trial and
acquittal) 28, 159, 170–
4, 202, 214
Sumner, Colin 22, 179
Sumner, William Graham
224
surgical practice (United
States) 197

Sutley, Joyce 101
Swartz, Donald 48,50
Swedlo, Mavis 142
Sweet, Lois 57

Taffel, S. 121
Taylor, Ian 40
teamwork 26, 99–100
teenage pregnancies 106–7
Tew, Marjorie 126–7
Thacker, Stephen 121
Thames Valley University
99, 203. See also mid-
wifery education
Thompson, E.P. 45, 52,
135
Thompson, Paul 78
Thunhurst, Colin 21
Tonkin, Roger 12, 128–9
traditional birth atten-
dants (TBAS) 74–5, 83–
93, 154–5
traditional birth culture
74, 160
transfer to hospital 28–9,
56, 120; from birth cen-
tres 145
Treichler, Paula 61, 131,
193
trial of labour 159, 181
Tuna, Nancy 76
Turk, Austin 47
Twaddle, Andrew 21
twins 56, 129
Tyson, Holliday 16, 90,
129–30

Ursel, Jane 60, 178–9

vacuum extraction, 20,
127
vaginal birth after caesarean (VBAC) 109–10,
136, 149, 164–5
Van Wagner, Vicki 56,
183, 193
Velimirovic, Helga 90
Ventre, Fran 144
Victorian Order of Nurses
(VON) 80, 192